JAN 19 2012

WITHDRAWN

W9-BDT-499

A Gift for

_____

Presented by

_____

Health...

The Reader's Digest VERSION

Health...

The Reader's Digest VERSION

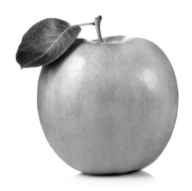

Easy ways to feel better and live longer

Joe Kita
and the staff of READER'S DIGEST magazine

Reader's
Digest

The Reader's Digest Association, Inc.
New York, NY/Montreal

Menasha Public Library
Menasha WI 54952
(920) 967-5166

Copyright © 2012 The Reader's Digest Association, Inc.

All rights reserved. Unauthorized reproduction, in any manner, is prohibited.

Reader's Digest is a registered trademark of The Reader's Digest Association, Inc.

Library of Congress Cataloging-in-Publication Data

Kita, Joe.

Health-- the Reader's digest version : great advice, simply put / by Joe Kita and
the staff of Reader's digest magazine. -- 1st ed.

   p. cm.

ISBN 978-1-60652-364-3

1. Health. 2. Nutrition. 3. Exercise. 4. Sleep. 5. Health promotion. 6. Self-care, Health. I. Title.

RA776.K59 2011

613.2--dc23

2011035080

We are committed to both the quality of our products and the service we provide our customers.
We value your comments, so please feel free to contact us.

   The Reader's Digest Association, Inc.
   Editor in Chief, Books & Home Entertainment
   44 South Broadway
   White Plains, NY 10601

For more Reader's Digest products and information, visit our website:

   www.readersdigest.com (in the United States)
   www. readersdigest.ca (in Canada)

Printed in the United States of America

1 3 5 7 9 10 8 6 4 2

NOTE TO OUR READERS

We pledge that the information and advice inside *Health... The Reader's Digest Version* has
been checked carefully for accuracy and is supported by leading health experts and up-to-
date research. However, each person's health and healing regimens are unique. Even the best
information should not be substituted for, or used to alter, medical therapy without your doctor's
advice. For a specific health problem, consult your physician for guidance.

"I don't want to get to the end of my life and find that I just lived the length of it. I want to have lived the width of it as well."

DIANE ACKERMAN, *AUTHOR*

"When it comes to eating right and exercising, there is no 'I'll start tomorrow.' Tomorrow is disease."

TERRI GUILLEMETS, *ANTHOLOGIST*

"The greatest wealth is health."

VIRGIL, *ROMAN POET*

"If you break a leg, don't come running to me."

CONNIE KITA, *MY MOTHER*

Contents

INTRODUCTION

When I was a boy, Dr. Rutledge was our family physician. He worked out of a small, homey brick office in Fountain Hill, Pennsylvania, with a wondrous aquarium in the waiting room that made it seem like you were never waiting very long. He worked in shirtsleeves without gloves and smelled like Clubman hair tonic. His nurses greeted us by name with genuine smiles, and I can't remember Dr. Rutledge ever making a referral; he fixed everything right there. And when your diagnosis was complete, he personally presented you—whether child or adult—with a Charms lollipop.

Now, some forty years later, my family has half a dozen doctors, even though we're all healthy. We have two general practitioners, a cardiologist, a dermatologist, an ob-gyn, plus

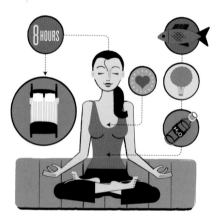

we occasionally see a nurse practitioner at the clinic in our local supermarket. The waiting rooms are all unadorned and interminable, staffed by people in lab coats smelling of hand sanitizer and latex. We're recognized by our files, not our faces. And the receptionist's first words are always, "Can I see your insurance card?"

Should one of us ever get really sick and have to "negotiate" the healthcare system, I'm warned we'll need to be our own advocates because things are so complex. Indeed, I've stopped trying to decipher the bills I'm sent. And lollipops? Well, those spike blood sugar and promote obesity, you know.

Having been a health journalist for thirty years, I worry that patients are losing their patience. Most people nowadays are so overwhelmed by the medical system and its costs, not to mention the bombardment of so much contradictory health and nutrition information by the media, that they're at the brink of inaction. Staying

Staying healthy shouldn't cause you to stress. Here is simple, empowering advice for making health easy—even pleasurable—to maintain.

healthy has become a source of stress rather than satisfaction.

That's why *Reader's Digest* has decided to do what it does best—gather and condense the most vital information on the topic of health and present it in a way that educates, enlightens, and empowers you. Although not designed to replace professional medical care, it is intended to simplify it. On the following pages, you'll find succinct, practical, straightforward advice on seventy essential facets of health, fitness, nutrition, and overall well-being. From snoring to skin cancer, cholesterol to cold sores, weight loss to healthcare costs...it's all here.

So turn the page and step into *our* office. The staff is friendly, there's no waiting, and proof of insurance isn't even required. And although we couldn't include a lollipop in the package, we guarantee you'll leave feeling this is one challenge you have unquestionably licked.

JOE KITA

Living well...

Instead of viewing life as a big-box discount store, where quantity is the driving force, it's time to start looking at it as a boutique shop, where quality is paramount. As evidenced at nursing homes nationwide, it's not the number of days in your life that matters but the amount of life in those days. All the advice in this section—from lowering stress to boosting energy to making love last—is designed to do just that. If living well is an art, consider this your foundational course.

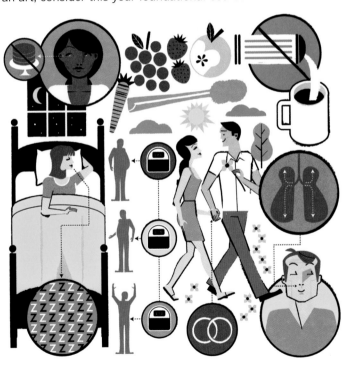

Sleep great
tonight (and every night)

If physicians took the time to pinpoint the cause of disease, the words "lack of sleep" would appear on many death certificates. Heart disease, stroke, diabetes, obesity, depression, even cancer are linked to not getting adequate rest—something of which 50 percent of Americans are guilty. Experts now estimate that the significantly sleep-deprived have a poorer quality of life and a 20 percent greater risk of death than the well rested. If you're tossing and turning, here's how to finally rest easy.

8 HOURS

Calculate and commit
For every two hours of wakefulness, you need one hour of sleep. So if you're up for sixteen hours, you should be down for eight. Do the math, and remember that sleep debt is cumulative. If you're not meeting your quota during the week, catch up on the weekend. Once you know how much rest you require, prioritize it. Sleeping is not a sign of laziness; it's the simplest, most important thing you can do for better health.

Set a caffeine deadline
This should generally be ten hours before bedtime. Caffeine has a half-life of about six hours, which means that 50 percent of what's ingested at noon is in your system at 6:00 P.M., and half of that still lingers at midnight. So the earlier you have your last jolt, the better. And this includes caffeinated teas, sodas, even chocolate.

Exercise regularly

Thirty minutes of moderate daily exercise produces feel-good hormones called endorphins that promote and deepen sleep. (Just avoid exercising within three hours of bedtime.)

Eat early and light

Allow four hours for digestion prior to bed, and make dinner the lightest meal of the day. Likewise, have your nightcap three hours before bed in order to give your body time to metabolize the alcohol.

LIVING UNDER THE INFLUENCE

>> After seventeen to nineteen hours without sleep, your brain activity is similar to someone with a blood alcohol content of 0.05. (The legal limit for intoxication in the United States is 0.08.)

Prepare the bat cave

Your bedroom should be dark, cool, and quiet. Block all ambient light, including the illuminated face of your alarm clock (turn it toward the wall). Set the temperature to 65°F (18°C) and use cotton pajamas and sheets. Keep TVs and computers out of the bedroom, and mask any neighborhood noise with the continuous low hum of a fan or a radio set between stations.

Flush

When you go to the bathroom for the final time, spend a few extra minutes writing your worries on a piece of tissue. Then throw it in the bowl and flush. There now, your mind is clear. Pleasant dreams....

Lose weight
for good

The reason most diets fail is because they require us to give up the foods we love. Still, we vow to be strong, bravely resist for weeks, and then, in a moment of weakness, we succumb to a craving, our diet disintegrates, and eventually we rebound to an even higher weight. If this sounds familiar, you should know there's a way to break this cycle and lose weight for good *without* swearing off your favorite foods.

Rather than changing *what* you eat, the secret is changing *how* you eat it, say the scientists behind the Small Plate Movement, an organization dedicated to getting families and restaurants to return to more sane food-portion sizes. These ideas might seem trivial, but by eating a little less at every meal, you will steadily return to your more natural weight.

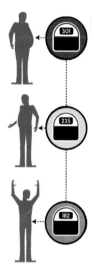

Switch from dinner to salad plates

Researchers at Cornell University found that switching to 8-inch plates from 10.4-inch plates (and, of course, not indulging in seconds) reduced calorie consumption by about 20 percent per meal. Not only does a smaller-diameter plate hold less food, it also creates an illusion of plenty by appearing full. This tricks the mind into feeling satisfied.

Choose smaller bowls

In a study published in the *American Journal of Preventive Medicine*, people who served themselves ice cream in 17-ounce bowls ate 31 percent less than those using bowls holding twice as much. And again, they didn't feel cheated, because the portion appeared relatively substantial.

Use a smaller spoon

The people in the study who were given a 2-ounce spoon ingested nearly 15 percent less than those using 3-ouncers. When small bowls *and* small spoons were used, 57 percent less ice cream was consumed without anyone feeling shortchanged. Something else might be at work, too. Since there's about a 20-minute lag between when your belly is full and the point at which your brain recognizes it, slowing your eating with smaller utensils helps you savor food more, causing you to naturally bridge that gap and eat less.

Select a small glass

Using short, wide drinking glasses typically results in about 20 percent less liquid being consumed compared to tall, skinny ones. Keep this in mind when drinking juice, soda, and alcohol.

Run with this concept

The possibilities for downsizing your dinnerware (and yourself!) are endless. For instance, use smaller serving utensils in casserole dishes. Set out smaller knives to spread cream cheese and butter. Swirl pasta around a smaller fork. Cut your food into tinier pieces. Buy kid-size snack packages.... To win the war on big, think small.

THE KEY QUESTION Before embarking on any diet, ask yourself this: Can I eat this way for the rest of my life? If the answer is no, then don't even start. Although subsisting on cabbage soup or mail-order diet meals may help you lose weight short-term, you'll inevitably tire of such restrictions. To be successful long-term, a diet shouldn't be a diet; it should be a lifestyle.

Avoid home
health traps

You fret about catching the latest media-hyped disease or whether your food is chemical-free, but one of the biggest threats to your family's health is right under your roof. Believe it or not, "home sweet home" is responsible for 20,000 deaths and 21 million medical visits annually. Instead of cleaning the toilets this weekend (admit it, you were looking for an excuse), here are the five biggest threats to address.

Keeping everybody upright

Falls are the leading cause of home injury and death, especially among children and older adults. So wipe out slipperiness in your house. Secure shaky railings, put nonslip strips in tubs and under throw rugs, clear off stairs, install nightlights in bedroom and bath areas, put guards or locks on toddlers' windows, spread fresh mulch around play areas, and replace those old step stools and ladders Grandpa gave you.

Protecting against poisoning

Secure anything that can be accidentally ingested (medications, vitamins, cleaning liquids, your brother's home brew...). Just in case, program the poison control hotline (1-800-222-1222) into everybody's phones. But pills and fluids aren't the only potential poisons. Carbon monoxide can be emitted from gas fireplaces, woodstoves, and other fuel-burning devices. Since it's odorless and deadly, install CO detectors near bedrooms.

Preventing fires and burns

Assuming all your fire extinguishers and smoke detectors are working, here are two things to check that most people overlook. Open and push down on your oven door. If the entire stove tips forward, call an appliance service to secure it. Next, inspect your water heater for signs of deterioration and leakage. It's one of the most dangerous appliances in the house, according to home inspectors, because it can explode. The temperature should also be set no higher than 120°F (49°C).

Breathing easy

Dive into the kids' toy chest and do the toilet paper–tube test. Anything small enough to fit through one is a choking hazard for children under five. Next, remove all pillows, blankets, and toys from the baby's crib—these are suffocation risks, as is putting the little guy to sleep on his chest or side. As for better air quality in your home, wage war on dust by sweeping often, use synthetic doormats (they don't get moldy), keep an eye on bathroom mold, and keep windows open as much as possible. Truth is, outdoor air is usually cleaner than indoor air.

Staying afloat

If you have a pool, spa, or pond, make sure they're adequately protected and/or equipped with floats. Suction from drains can be particularly hazardous, so install safety guards. Being certified in CPR is also a great skill. Contact your local Red Cross chapter to enroll in a thirty-minute citizen class.

ARE YOU SMOKING WITHOUT REALIZING IT? Smoking is the leading cause of lung cancer. No surprise there. But were you aware that radon, an odorless and invisible gas, is the runner-up? It's even more deadly than secondhand smoke. Radon comes from decaying uranium, which exists naturally in the earth in many parts of the world. It can work its way through home foundations and even into water. Buy a test kit at a home-supply store or visit epa.gov/radon to learn more.

Brave a craving

L ife is one big constant crave. Whether it's food, beauty, money, gadgets, sex, or status, we are an incredibly rich society that somehow still needs everything. For proof, just look in your closet, garage, or rental unit at the U-Store-It Village. Or even more troubling, look at your middle in the mirror. In fact, let's start there. If you can learn to control your food cravings, which are the most frequent and irresistible of all, you'll be on your way to resisting other temptations as well.

Determine what you're really hungry for

The next time you get a craving, ask yourself if you're stressed, frustrated, sad, or bored. If so, then you're eating to fill an emotional void rather than a physical one. Try keeping a "desire diary" for a week. Whenever a craving strikes, note your mood. If stress turns out to be your trigger, exercise more to relieve the pressure. If it's loneliness that's driving you to the Doritos bag, call someone or join a social network such as Facebook or Meetup. Remember also that true hunger is easy to satisfy; any food will do. But emotional hunger usually manifests in desires for specific things like chocolate, ice cream, or Burger King.

Get off the energy roller coaster

The second biggest cause of cravings is a diet with too much refined carbohydrate. This causes drops in blood sugar that prompt hunger. For instance, if you have a bagel or donut for breakfast, you'll get a nice jolt of energy from the sugar, but by mid-morning you'll be craving another. To stabilize energy levels and appetite, eat more protein and fiber. Tomorrow have eggs and whole-wheat toast or a bowl of fiber-rich cereal with nuts and see if you can easily make it to lunch.

Stay hydrated

Many people think they're hungry when they're actually thirsty. To test if a food craving is genuine, drink a glass of water and wait a few minutes to see if it subsides. At the very least, you'll be better hydrated.

Distract yourself

Taste buds have a very short attention span. Instead of instantly giving into a craving, pop a mint, brush your teeth, check e-mail, call a friend, or just wait five minutes. In most cases, you'll find you weren't really hungry.

15 » The number of minutes of walking it takes to successfully stifle a chocolate craving. Skeptical? Try it. If the urge doesn't subside, then indulge yourself. At least you'll already have burned a good chunk of the calories.

Redo your kitchen

Put all your crave foods on the lowest shelf in the back of the fridge or in the cabinet you need a step stool to reach. This will give you more time to think before you eat.

Hang on to your hair

We all know that guys often lose their hair. But here's an interesting statistic: A man's age gives a good approximation of the probability that he has started balding. For example, at age fifty, chances that you've started balding are around 50 percent. Less known, and more frightening, is that about 55 percent of women experience hair loss at some point in their lives. Often it starts during menopause. Although hair loss is mostly an inherited condition resulting from a complex gene interaction, there are some simple things you can do to avoid triggering it sooner and retaining more of what you have longer.

Save on product

Despite how Rihanna makes it seem when she dances, hair is not a living thing. Once it pops out of your head, it's dead. So for retention purposes, it's better to focus on what's happening below the surface, or inside the hair follicle. Most people get that backward.

Learn to relax

Stress, whether it's ongoing anxiety from work or a traumatic event like the death of a friend, can prompt hereditary hair loss to start sooner—a condition called shedding. Manage your stress better by adopting a yoga mindset. Here's the mantra: *I can't control what happens, but I can control my reaction to what happens*. Just that little shift in thinking can make a big difference. Try it.

Stop dieting

Hair follicles, like all living organisms, need good nutrition to function. So don't starve yours by going on restrictive fad diets. The body interprets these as another form of stress. Instead, control weight with exercise and smarter eating. Vegetarians should make sure to meet RDAs for protein and iron, since deficiencies in either can cause hair loss. (Forget special hair vitamins, though; there's no clinical proof they work.)

Keep the blood flowing

Hair follicles also require good circulation to flourish. Regular aerobic exercise strengthens the heart so it can pump more blood up there. Likewise, keep your arteries lean and flexible by eating a low-fat, fiber-rich diet and not smoking.

DON'T WORRY, IT'S NORMAL

50 to 100 » The average number of hairs per day the average person loses from his or her scalp.

Assess your meds

Certain medications and supplements can trigger hair loss. Among them are antidepressants, beta-blockers, steroids, and even too much vitamin A. If you notice thinning after you start popping a new pill, check the side effects and discuss alternatives with your doctor.

Wear a hat

A bad sunburn on the scalp releases an inflammatory compound called superoxide that causes follicles to shut down. Contrary to popular belief, hats don't prompt hair loss; they protect against it.

Consult a hair doctor

The next time you have a skin screening, ask your dermatologist to assess the condition of your scalp and hair. If there's trouble, she can do a scalp biopsy to determine if it's temporary or longer lasting, and you can discuss regrowth options, such as oral finasteride for men or topical minoxidil, which works for both men and women.

Be a smarter
supermarket shopper

I f your supermarket trips have become super-long because
of all the label reading and brand comparison you're
doing, it's time to streamline your strategy. Here
are some quick ways to determine whether a
product is healthful or hyped, so you can get
on with your life.

Forget about package claims

Terms such as "natural," "good source of...," "low
fat," and even "whole grain" are all unregulated marketing
buzzwords. For example, a product may be labeled "made with
real fruit juice" yet contain just a small amount. Or it can say
"zero trans fats," "fat-free," or "sugar-free" and still legally contain up to 0.5 grams per serving of each, which can add up if the
serving size is relatively small. So never grab anything based
solely on marketing claims.

Scan the ingredients

Nina Planck, a real-food expert and author, recommends paying
more attention to a product's ingredient list than its Nutrition
Facts panel. She contends that counting calories, grams of protein, and other nutrients takes the enjoyment out of eating by
making it a confusing science. Instead, when deciding between
brands, she simply chooses the one with the fewest and most
recognizable ingredients. Doing so usually guarantees she's
buying food that's "whole," or closer to its original state, and
thus more healthful.

Beware these words

If, among the ingredients, you spot high-fructose corn syrup
(or other words ending in "ose," such as maltose, dextrose, and

sucrose), hydrogenated oils, artificial flavors and colors, or anything you can't pronounce, put the item back on the shelf. Corn syrup and other added sugars have been linked to obesity and its many woes, while hydrogenated oils and chemical additives can promote cancers.

Check a few key facts
Two-thirds of shoppers read nutrition panels, but fewer than half understand them. So don't try to digest the whole thing. Instead, focus on three statistics: 1) saturated fat (should be less than 7 percent of total daily value); 2) sodium (should be less than 300 mg per serving); and 3) serving size (should not be so small that you can easily eat three or more at a sitting, which multiplies all values accordingly).

Shop naked
The best foods are those that don't come dressed in packages. Fresh fruits and vegetables, for example, don't need any hype or analysis, because they are what they are, plain and simple. Fill your basket with them.

LET YOUR PHONE MAKE THE CALL There are more and more mobile phone apps that enable shoppers to scan a product's bar code and receive an instant healthfulness rating (plus recommendations for smarter choices, if necessary). Popular ones include Fooducate, GoodGuide, and CerealScan. Make sure, however, that the app you choose is not marketed or sponsored by a food manufacturer, which may make it biased.

Best 10 minute workout:
Sun salutations

It's better to do a little exercise a lot rather than a lot of exercise a little. The second approach will get you injured, while the first one—even if it's just ten minutes per day—will eventually make you fit, slim, and healthy. Yoga classes traditionally begin with a series of ten postures linked in a continuous flowing motion that elevates heart rate, boosts metabolism, and stretches and strengthens just about every muscle in the body. It's called a Sun Salutation. Start your day with ten minutes' worth and enjoy the benefits.

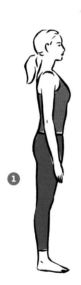

1. *Stand tall at the front of your mat with both feet touching and arms at your sides. Inhale and exhale deeply through the nose three times.*

2. *Inhale while extending and raising both arms overhead until palms meet. Gaze up.*

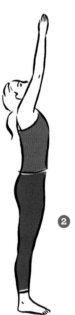

3. *Exhale and fold forward bringing your chest toward your knees and your head toward your toes. Hands should rest on the floor, ankles, or knees.*

4. *Inhale and, without moving your hands, come up halfway, lengthening your spine and directing your gaze out in front.*

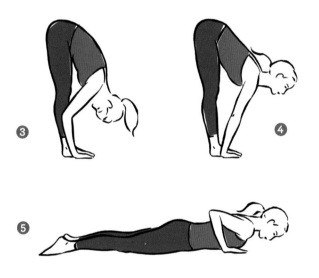

5. *Exhale and step back with one foot and then the other until you're in a high plank position. Keep elbows tucked, lower to the floor, just as if finishing a push-up.*

6. Inhale and straighten your arms while rolling onto the tops of your feet. Legs are extended behind as the chest approaches a 90-degree angle with the floor. This is called up-dog.

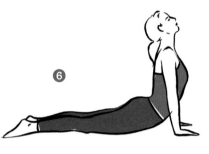

7. Exhale and push back into down-dog. You should resemble an upside-down V, with fingers spread wide and heels on or pushing toward the floor. Let your head dangle. Hold the pose for five complete breaths.

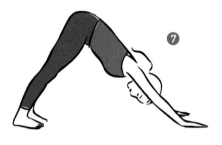

8. Inhale while stepping one foot and then the other between your hands. Lengthen the spine and look ahead as in step 4.

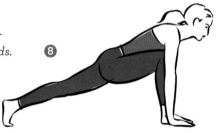

9. *Exhale and fold forward as in step 3.*

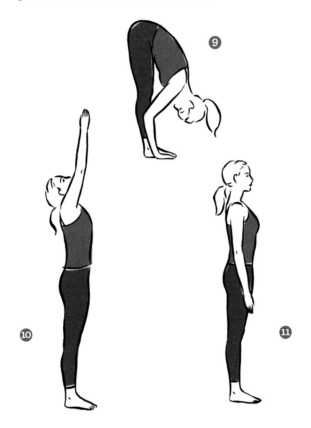

10. *Inhale while coming up and raising both arms as in step 2.*

11. *Lower arms back to the start position, take three breaths, and repeat.*

Find your
ideal exercise

Exercise is the answer. When done regularly, it burns fat, brightens mood, fights disease, and even makes you more attractive. So why don't more people embrace it? Because they haven't found the exercise they were designed for, both physically and psychologically. If your basement is a jungle of discarded infomercial gear, if you've quit more gyms than a pastry chef has eaten cupcakes, here's how to finally find your "soul game."

Match your personality
If you're an extrovert, then pedaling a stationary bike in your basement or watching exercise DVDs on your TV isn't going to satisfy you for long. Better to sign up for Zumba or join a team in training for a charity run or ride. Conversely, if you're a loner, then the solitary space that walking, running, or a home gym affords should appeal to you more.

Match your body type
If you're naturally big-boned, then running and other high-impact activities will never be comfortable (or healthy) for you. Better to choose a weight-bearing exercise like spinning or swimming. Likewise, if you're smallish, then being in a weight room with a bunch of Amazons will forever make you feel inferior. Try a more vigorous style of yoga, like Ashtanga, to tone your muscles.

Regress
To further hone in on your ideal exercise, think about the activities you enjoyed as a kid. Maybe you loved skipping rope,

pedaling a bike, or hiking and exploring in the woods. Revisit them. Chances are, even decades later you'll still experience the same joy.

Banish the word "workout"

The power of suggestion is...well, powerful. Every time you refer to exercise as *working* out, you're creating a negative association in your subconscious. Instead, start thinking of it as playtime or recess (mark it on your calendar as such) and see if you don't anticipate it more.

Dabble

Many people find they have an ideal exercise *type* rather than just one perfect pastime. This is good. If you discover you feed off the energy of group classes, then don't limit yourself to just one brand or instructor. Change up weekly or monthly. The variety will keep your mind and body fresh.

Consider one more alternative

Your ideal exercise may be much broader than you originally thought. Researchers are finding that being active throughout the day (housework, gardening, running errands) is better for overall well-being and even weight loss than confining activity to an hour or so and being sedentary the rest of the day. So if an exercise you try doesn't seem to click, then just be more active.

GIVE IT THE TEST You'll know you've found your soul game when the time you spend doing it becomes timeless. You'll look at your watch and be stunned an hour (or more!) has passed. This is known as flow, or being in the sweet spot. Relish it.

Beat fatigue,
boost energy

Ever wonder why zombies are so popular nowadays? We have a theory. Maybe it's because watching them stagger around makes us feel well rested by comparison. Indeed, we have become a Zombie Nation in ways beyond entertainment. James B. Maas, PhD, a Cornell University sleep researcher, estimates as many as 70 million Americans are chronically sleep deprived, which costs the country $66 billion annually in lost productivity, accidents, and illness. Frightening, isn't it? Here's how to leave the ranks of the living dead.

Pay off your sleep debt
Most people don't realize that sleep debt is cumulative. If you lose an hour or two a few nights in a row, you won't feel fresh until you make that downtime up. Adults need seven to nine hours of sleep per night, or 56 to 63 hours per week, to stay healthy and energized. Keep a weekly tally.

Become less chemically dependent
Resorting to caffeine, nicotine, alcohol, or other stimulants to overcome fatigue is a short-term solution with debilitating long-term effects. Not only can you develop unhealthful dependencies on these substances, they can also interfere with sleep, which defeats the purpose of taking them in the first place.

Exercise to energize
Although it sounds contradictory, expending energy gives you *more* energy. This is due to the fatigue-fighting, mood-enhancing brain chemicals released during physical activity. Skeptical? Try this: The next time you need a pick-me-up, go for a walk or do some calisthenics. The exercise doesn't even have to be vigorous to make you feel more alert.

Eat more often and more densely

Eating lots of unrefined carbohydrate, like white bread, rice, and pasta, is akin to trying to keep a fire burning with newsprint. There's an immediate flare-up, but the flames subside quickly. Better to stoke yourself with a steady supply of denser, longer-burning, complex carbohydrate (whole grains, beans, fruits, and vegetables) and lean protein. Even better, eat five or six smaller meals per day rather than the usual two or three. More frequent, more diverse eating will also supply a wider range of nutrients, which will help correct any deficiencies that may be compounding your tiredness.

Keep water in the tank

Being just 2 percent underhydrated can make you act and feel older. For a sharp mind, smooth skin, better health, and fluid movement, you need water. But forget about the old eight-times-eight rule (eight 8-ounce glasses of water daily). Healthy eaters, it turns out, get all the water they need from what they routinely eat and drink (that includes tea and coffee but not alcoholic beverages). If you're thirsty, though, drink up. And if you've worked up a sweat exercising, are in a hot climate, or are taking medications, you may need to drink more than usual.

HAVE A NAP-A-LATTE TO GO There is nothing more naturally energy-boosting than a nap of 10 to 30 minutes. Dipping into just the first couple stages of sleep refreshes and restores alertness. Don't sleep any longer than that, though, or you'll awaken groggier than when you started, a condition called sleep inertia.

For those times when you need to power through, here's a recipe from sleep expert Michael Breus, PhD. He calls it a "nap-a-latte": Drink a lukewarm-to-cold cup of drip coffee (it has the most caffeine), then close your eyes for 20 to 25 minutes. "You'll get just enough sleep to reduce fatigue, and when the caffeine kicks in, you'll be good for another four hours."

Be your own
massage therapist

Studies show that regular massage is one of the simplest yet most effective ways to lower stress and boost mood. But it's an expensive habit if done by a pro, and unfortunately, most spouses will only indulge you after much begging and negotiating. So it's time to take matter into your own hands, so to speak. Here are our favorite self-massage tricks and techniques to finally get you rubbed the right way.

Let the good times roll
If you think of your muscles as dough that kneads to be relaxed, then you'll grasp the concept behind high-density foam rollers. Generally about 5 inches (13 cm) thick and 1 to 3 feet (30 to 91 cm) long, they're especially good for lying on and massaging a sore back or legs. For a cheaper alternative try a swimming pool noodle, rolling pin, or fresh paint roller.

Smile constantly at work
Fill a zipper-seal bag with marbles and put it on the floor under your desk. Periodically remove your shoes and roll the stress away. (It's even more indulgent during long staff meetings.)

Slip into some new beans
Fill your house slippers with a thin layer of small, uncooked beans and enjoy a foot massage while you clean. Bonus: If your spouse ticks you off by refusing to help, make chili.

Turn the bathroom into a spa
Water massage is called hydrotherapy. If you have a whirlpool bath, position your lower back, the soles of your feet, or any other cranky muscle in front of a jet. Likewise, let the spray from

your showerhead gently massage your scalp, face, neck, and shoulders.

Use the old sock-and-rice trick

If you haven't done this before, you're in for a treat. Find an old athletic sock (but no holes!), fill it with rice, then securely tie the top. Throw in the microwave and heat for 60 to 90 seconds. Lay the sock on any sore muscles for incredible relief as the rice contours to your body. It's particularly nice around the back of your neck. Don't empty the sock afterward; use it over and over.

Have a ball

Just about any type of ball can be a self-massage tool. Roll a golf ball around with your tootsies, soothe sore shoulders and thighs with a baseball, or stuff two tennis balls into a sock. Then tie the end and use the leverage from a floor or wall to roll them along your spine.

Train your pet to walk on your back

This works best with a small dog (as opposed to a canary or Doberman). Lie facedown on the floor while a friend repeats a command such as "Rubdown!" and uses a treat to entice the pet to walk around on your back. In time all you'll need to do is lie down, repeat the command, and let Magic Paws take over. Cats also make great heating pads. Train yours to curl up on your back and you'll be purring in no time.

DONATE YOUR BODY TO SCIENCE Visit massageschools.net to see if there's a massage-therapy school near you. If so, call to see if the students need any volunteer bodies to work on. If so, you may be able to score a massage for free or at a deep discount.

Decide if
organic is worth it

Sticker shock used to be confined to new cars and the occasional rude T-shirt. Not anymore. If you're like most shoppers, you're probably aghast at the price of organic alternatives in the supermarket. If you're confused as to whether organic is worth the expense, here's some guidance.

Don't assume it's good for you

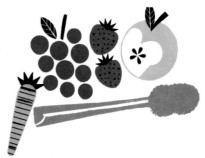

In the last few years "organic" has become just another marketing buzzword. There's now organic cake mix, hot dogs, ice cream, soda, and even lard and tobacco. It's an effective word, too. Many people believe, falsely, that products featuring the label are healthier, or lower in calories, than their non-organic counterparts. That's simply not true. So if you're out to lose weight and get fit, don't misinterpret eating organic as the way to do it.

Don't assume it's more nutritious

A review published in the *American Journal of Clinical Nutrition* examined 50 years of organic-versus-conventional-food studies and concluded: "There is no evidence of a difference in nutrient quality." What you're essentially buying when you choose organic is a pesticide- and chemical-free product that's better for the environment and less toxic for your body, not one with more vitamins and minerals.

Don't assume it tastes better

There's little research to support the notion that organic tastes superior; any perceived difference is probably a case of justifying expense by using mind over platter. That said, *we* certainly think we taste the difference between locally grown produce bought the day after it was harvested and food raised on super-farms and shipped across the country. But that might have nothing to do with organics.

Clean up the largest part of your diet

If buying organic is important to you, there's no need to revamp your entire diet and blow your food budget. Many lower-priced, non-organic foods aren't much different from their organic counterparts. To help you decide which organics to buy, draw a food pyramid for your family. Put those things eaten most at the bottom and those consumed least up top. Then, as food scientist and nutritionist Mary Ellen Camire, PhD, suggests, direct most of your organic food dollars at what's foundational. For instance, if you're a meat-eggs-and-potato family then buy organic there, where it will have the most impact.

Know the lingo

All organic products are not created equal. There is special terminology designated by the USDA for food labeling. If it says "100% organic," then all ingredients (except water and salt) are exactly that. "Organic" means it contains at least 95 percent organically produced ingredients. And "made with organic ingredients" means it contains at least 70 percent. The green-and-white "USDA Organic" seal can only legally be used with the first two designations. Produce advertised as "organically grown" must also meet strict USDA standards for growing, handling, and processing. Incidentally, the term natural is not interchangeable with organic and is, in fact, not even USDA regulated.

Grow your own

If you want superior taste and nutrition without the expense and confusion, plant an organic garden. Just-picked produce is the most healthful food of all, plus you'll have the added chutz-pah of knowing you grew it.

WHEN TO SPEND, WHEN TO SAVE Each year the Environmental Working Group analyzes the pesticide residue on commercially sold produce and recommends where your organic food dollars are best spent. Here's the latest list:

Buy Organic

▸▸ Apples

▸▸ Celery

▸▸ Strawberries

▸▸ Peaches

▸▸ Spinach

▸▸ Nectarines (imported)

▸▸ Grapes (imported)

▸▸ Sweet bell peppers

▸▸ Potatoes

▸▸ Blueberries (domestic)

▸▸ Lettuce

▸▸ Kale/collard greens

Buy Regular

▸▸ Onions

▸▸ Sweet corn

▸▸ Pineapples

▸▸ Avocado

▸▸ Asparagus

▸▸ Sweet peas

▸▸ Mangoes

▸▸ Eggplant

▸▸ Cantaloupe (domestic)

▸▸ Kiwi

▸▸ Cabbage

▸▸ Watermelon

▸▸ Sweet potatoes

▸▸ Grapefruit

▸▸ Mushrooms

PERSONAL N●TES

{ How can I live **more organically?** }

Live to 100+

It's not that difficult. The consensus of 100 doctors we polled is that at least 60 percent of chronic disease can be avoided by doing 12 simple things. In fact, studies of identical twins, who share the same genes but not the same habits or environment, suggest DNA dictates only 25 to 33 percent of life expectancy. But the following checklist isn't just a prescription for living long; it's your ticket to living well. And it's never too late to start.

1. **Stop smoking**
   Four years after doing so, your chance of having a heart attack falls to that of someone who's never smoked. After 10 years your lung cancer risk drops to nearly that of a nonsmoker.

2. **Exercise daily**
   Thirty minutes of light activity is all that's necessary. Three 10-minute walks will do it.

3. **Eat five servings of fresh fruit/vegetables daily**
   These are full of antioxidants—the Army Rangers of protective nutrients. You want platoons of them deployed in your bloodstream at all times.

4. **Get screened**
   Elsewhere in this book we list the best health tests to get at different stages of life. Follow them.

5. **Get plenty of sleep**
   For most adults that means eight to nine hours every night. This is when your body's immune system reloads.

6. **Take a daily low-dose aspirin**
   Heart attack, stroke, even cancer… Just a single 81-mg tablet per day appears to fight them all. But consult your doctor before you start, in case it conflicts with other medication.

7. ***Know your blood pressure***
   It's not called the silent killer because our lives need more drama. Keep yours around 120/80.

8. ***Stay connected***
   Loneliness is another form of stress. Friends, family, and furry pets supply vitamin F.

9. ***Cut back on saturated fat***
   It's the raw material your body uses for producing bad (LDL) cholesterol.

10. ***Get help for depression***
    As they say in *The Sopranos,* depression is rage turned inward. It's self-destructive. In fact, when tacked onto diabetes or heart disease, it increases risk of early death by as much as 30 percent.

11. ***Manage stress***
    The doctors we surveyed claim that living with uncontrolled stress is more destructive to physical and mental health than being 30 pounds overweight.

12. ***Have a higher purpose***
    As one physician advised, "Strive to achieve something bigger than yourself." Whether this happens via church, community, or charity, when you give back, you also give to yourself.

BOCA BETTER BRACE ITSELF

71,991 ▶▶ Estimated number of centenarians in the United States in 2010

601,000 ▶▶ Projected number of centenarians in the United States in 2050, thanks both to better health care and people taking better care of themselves

Raise a
fit kid

One out of every three American kids is overweight or obese and destined for all the health woes that bestows. What has caused childhood obesity rates to triple in the last 30 years? Not McDonalds. Not Nintendo. It's parents and grandparents. We're the ones who teach, direct, inspire, and shape. But this is one responsibility we've dropped like a heavy weight. If you have a toddler who's become a waddler, or a teen who wears big jeans because they're practical rather than trendy, here's how to get 'em in shape.

Lead by example

Children learn by watching more than listening. So if your only exercise is Cheez Doodle biceps curls, don't expect them to grow up any differently. Prioritize working out and eating smart, and they will, too. It's that simple.

Emphasize activity over dieting

Restrictive fad diets are physically and mentally damaging to kids, depriving them of essential nutrients for development and setting them up for failure because they aren't long-term solutions. It's better to promote fitness and weight loss by encouraging them to move more. Notice we didn't use the word "exercise." To a youngster exercise is activity minus the fun. So sneak more movement into everyday life by walking or pedaling rather than driving, and planning active vacations rather than sedentary ones. Buy bikes instead of gaming systems. Subscribe to being outside instead of Netflix. Be your family's activity coordinator.

Bring back home cookin'

Kids are swallowing 31 percent more calories, 56 percent more fats and oils, and 14 percent more sugars and sweeteners than they were 40 years ago. A major reason is because the average family spends about a third of its food budget at restaurants, where there's little control over what's ordered or how it's prepared. Save money and pounds by cooking more at home.

Improve snack quality

Forbidding kids to snack ultimately leads to candy caches in the toy chest. Instead, make fresh fruit more available and cut it up. Buy microwave popcorn instead of chips. And replace soda with fresh-brewed, mildly sweetened iced tea (or any of the other healthful drinks listed on page 58). Kids are lazy; they'll grab what's available.

Never use food as a carrot

Buying Junior a Happy Meal or chocolate bar every time he gets an A on his report card or scores a goal forever links fatty food with comfort in his subconscious. Instead, reward him verbally or with money (hey, this is America).

BRIBE 'EM! To give your gang more incentive to be active, create a reward system. Are the kids clamoring to go to Walt Disney World? Son wants a new skateboard? Make 'em earn it! Create a system that awards one point for each minute of activity, whether it's bicycling or taking out the recycling. Or buy everyone a pedometer and tally total steps each day. Keep track of everyone's progress on a kitchen whiteboard. By the time their goal is met, being more active will be a habit.

Make these health moves in
your 20s

What	When
Routine checks/exams	
Complete physical	Every 5 years
Blood pressure	At least once a year
Cholesterol	Every 5 years
Blood glucose	Every 3 years *(if at risk; ask your doctor)*
Eyesight	At least once this decade
Teeth	Twice yearly
Hearing	At least once this decade
Body mass index (BMI)	Annually
Skin cancer	Every 3 years
Testicular cancer	Monthly self-exam
Pelvic exam/Pap test	Annually for 3 years, then *(if normal)* every 2 to 3 years

Health... The Reader's Digest VERSION

This is when the foundation for future youth is laid. It's the decade for taking care of important long-term safeguards and cultivating good health habits. While it's not easy to prioritize health at such a seemingly invincible age, the steps taken now are no less important to eventual prosperity than starting a 401K.

Inoculations

Influenza	Annually
Hepatitis A	Once per lifetime *(if at risk, ask doctor)*
Hepatitis B	Once per lifetime *(if at risk, ask doctor)*
HPV (cervical cancer/genital warts)	Once per lifetime for women < age 26
Pneumonia	Once < age 64 *(if at risk, ask doctor)*
Meningitis	Once per lifetime *(if at risk, ask doctor)*
Chickenpox	Once per lifetime
Measles/mumps/rubella	Once < age 49
Tetanus-diphtheria	Once per decade
Whooping cough	Once per lifetime

General

Build strength.	Muscles are now at their developmental peak.
Line up good docs.	They'll be your lifetime advocates.
Do a family health history.	What killed Grandma could get you.

Never have a heart attack

That's quite a promise, we know. But University of Minnesota researchers estimate that nearly 90 percent of first-time heart attacks can be prevented. You already know about not smoking, avoiding saturated fat, reducing stress, and losing weight, but here are some other important cornerstones of heart health you should be building upon.

Treat your heart like a muscle
That's because it is one. And by exercising it regularly and aerobically, you can increase its size; extreme athletes have been shown to increase theirs by 30 to 40 percent. When you strengthen your heart, it's able to pump more blood with each stroke and doesn't need to beat as often overall. A lower pulse generally correlates with a healthier heart and a longer life. Swimmers, cross-country skiers, rowers, and cyclists tend to have the largest hearts.

Take your medicine
Cholesterol-lowering statins, blood pressure medication, and daily aspirin have all been proven safe and effective for reducing the risk of heart attack. Yet those Minnesota researchers found that most first-time heart-attack sufferers weren't taking advantage of them and, in most cases, may not even have been screened for cardiovascular disease. If you have a family history of heart trouble or other risk factors (overweight, smoker, stressed...), call to schedule a checkup with a cardiologist—*today.*

Add these items to your shopping list
Apples, almonds, avocados, bananas, barley, berries, broccoli, carrots, coffee (in moderation), kidney beans, kiwis, grape juice, lean beef, lentils, milk, mushrooms, oatmeal, olive oil, onions, papayas, pomegranate juice, red wine, spinach, sweet potatoes,

tea (green, white, black, oolong), tomatoes, turkey, walnuts, watermelon, wild salmon, and (yes!) dark chocolate. Because of the special nutrients (chiefly antioxidants and fiber) they contain, all these foods are extremely heart healthy. By the way, science now recommends getting nutrients naturally via food rather than in pill form. Our bodies don't seem to utilize most nutrients the same way when swallowed as supplements.

Live a life of "we," not "me"

According to Stephen Post, PhD, professor of preventive medicine at Stony Brook University, the more frequently a person uses "self-referencing" words, such as I, me, and my, the greater their risk of having a heart attack. Seems odd, but it turns out that emotional connection—not separateness—is good for the heart in more ways than one. Research shows that a strong support network of friends and family, along with a charitable and optimistic mindset, lowers stress, boosts immunity, and even hastens recovery if you ever do get sick.

THE TICKER

- ▶▶ **100,000** = number of times your heart beats in one day
- ▶▶ **35 million** = number of times your heart beats in one year
- ▶▶ **2.5 billion** = number of times your heart beats in a lifetime
- ▶▶ **6 quarts** = amount of blood in the human body
- ▶▶ **20 seconds** = time it takes for all that blood to circulate through the body
- ▶▶ **12,000 miles** = distance that blood travels in one day
- ▶▶ **1 million** = number of barrels of blood pumped in one lifetime
- ▶▶ **3** = number of supertankers those barrels would fill

Avoid food-borne illness

When you think of dangerous foods, chicken-fried steak and drive-thru megaburgers typically come to mind but they're not the only threat. That honor, according to the FDA, goes to 10 foods that seem surprisingly benign. In fact, you've probably eaten most of them this week. Here, in ascending order of risk, are the non-meat culprits for most of the 76 million cases of food-borne illness reported each year in the United States, along with how to avoid being victimized by each.

10 » Berries
Nooks and crannies provide hideouts for bad guys. Depending on the fruit's fragility, soak, spray, or scrub with fresh water. Avoid ordering in restaurants where the likelihood of a good cleaning is low.

9 » Sprouts
As with cigarettes and alcohol, these may soon sprout FDA warning labels because of how challenging they are to distribute safely and clean. Swear off them entirely.

8 » Tomatoes
Don't buy ones with splits or cracks (windows for salmonella) or eat them fresh at restaurants (48,000 outbreaks occur there). Otherwise, wash well in water.

7 » Ice cream
Soft-serve is particularly hazardous because bacterium often thrives in the dispensing machines. If you're making your own ice cream, try to use recipes that skip the raw egg.

6 » Cheese
As with ice cream, it's mostly the soft varieties that trouble stomachs. Brie, Camembert, feta, queso franco, and anything homemade should be approached with caution.

5 » **Potatoes**

Nana was right: Beware the potato salad. Forty percent of outbreaks involving spuds originate in restaurants and grocery delis because of improper storage.

4 » **Oysters**

These bivalves can contain the same family of bacterium as cholera. Slurp some soup as an appetizer instead.

3 » **Tuna**

Approximately 65 percent of illnesses from this fish can be traced back to restaurants. So if you're craving tuna salad or a nice filet, make it yourself and cook thoroughly.

2 » **Eggs**

Never eat raw or runny ones, and avoid indulging in eggs (or egg dishes) at breakfast buffets or catered events, where warming temperatures may be inadequate.

1 » **Leafy greens**

How can something so nutritious be atop a most-dangerous foods list? The simple reason is, greens often aren't washed properly, if at all. The FDA says to be particularly wary of restaurant salads and to always clean prepackaged supermarket greens even if the label says "prewashed."

WHAT NOT TO DO IF YOU'RE HIT... Something you ate turning your stomach? Skip the anti-diarrhea medication. You want that bug, whatever it is, out of you pronto. By resorting to Imodium or other similar medicines, you could slow its passage and worsen your condition. Most cases of food poisoning last less than 48 hours, during which time you should rest and stay hydrated. Anything beyond that needs a doctor's expertise.

Boost your immunity

If your mom was anything like ours, then staying healthy was a simple matter of "Don't get your feet wet!" and "Zip up your coat!" Although science disproved those two warnings long ago—along with "Someday your face will freeze like that!"—some of mom's favorite threats about avoiding impending death did turn out to be correct. To bolster your body's defense against germs and illness, listen to her for once.

"Don't be such a sourpuss!"

"Happier people are less likely to develop colds when exposed to cold viruses," says Sheldon Cohen, PhD, a professor of psychology at Carnegie Mellon University. Even the simple act of smiling fights infection.

"Go play outside!"

Regular exercise increases the number of disease-fighting cells patrolling the bloodstream. And if you exercise outdoors for 10 or 15 minutes before applying sunscreen, you'll also get an immunity-boosting dose of vitamin D (the sunshine vitamin), which is low in 50 percent of adults.

"Eat your vegetables!"

The brightest and deepest colored ones have the most antioxidants. But if stuff like spinach still makes you grimace, "hide" a nice assortment of them—plus health-ensuring onions, garlic, and tomatoes—in a pot of homemade vegetarian chili. Top each bowl with a dollop of probiotic-rich Greek yogurt. It's the new chicken soup.

"Be nice to your brother!"

Charitable acts raise levels of immunoglobulin A, an antibody in saliva that fights infection. In fact, just observing or considering generosity does it. When Harvard students watched a documentary of Mother Teresa ministering to the sick, they enjoyed the same effect.

"Go wash your hands!"

Despite how cliché it sounds, this is the single best thing you can do to stay healthy. Either use alcohol-based gels, or scrub for 20 seconds with soap and water. And then keep your fingers out of your mouth!

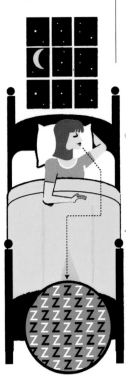

"It'll only hurt for a little while!"

Nearly 50,000 American adults die annually from diseases that could have easily, inexpensively, and painlessly been prevented with basic inoculations. See the decade-by-decade "Health Moves" sections throughout this book for what shots to get when.

"Go to bed already!"

Not getting the recommended seven and a half to nine hours of sleep per night raises your risk of colds, flu, obesity, diabetes, heart disease, and even cancer. As an example of just how important rest is to health, a University of Chicago study found that men with no risk factors for diabetes were in a pre-diabetic state after just one week of poor sleep. (See "Sleep Great Tonight and Every Night," page 12.)

SURPRISING THINGS YOU CAN CATCH It's not just the sniffles and pinkeye that are contagious. Apparently, so is…

▸▸ **Obesity** Adenovirus-36 is more likely to be found in the obese than the thin. And when lab animals are exposed to this virus, they begin gaining weight. Although more research is needed, the theory is that some viruses might infect cells and cause them to store fat.

▸▸ **Heart attack** Myocarditis is an inflammation of the heart muscle that can be triggered by a range of viral infections (cold, mononucleosis, measles, and HIV as well as bacterial infections.) If you have a stubborn illness, see a doctor before it works its way into your heart.

▸▸ **Divorce** According to research at the University of California, San Diego, the breakup of friends increases your chance of divorce by 147 percent. Psychologists call it "divorce clustering" and speculate that it encourages an if-they-can-so-can-I attitude.

▸▸ **Emotions** Other people's moods can infect yours. A study even quantified it: One sad friend doubles your chance of also becoming sad. And for each happy friend you have, your chance of personal happiness rises by 11 percent.

Lower your stress by
75 percent

You've heard the scary statistics—how millions fall victim to heart disease, stroke, and cancer every year. In fact, you're probably reading this book in the hopes of finding the key to minimizing your risk. Well, here it is: Lower your stress. Stress is a major underlying cause of disease and deterioration, both physical and mental. Yet in our misguided minds we've come to accept it as a normal part of modern life. While it's true that some stress is necessary for success (it pushes us), we're way over the healthy limit. Here are the simplest and best ways we've found to manage it.

Learn to say no
Much of stress is self-inflicted. It comes from being too nice and trying to do too much. To instantly cure yourself of this, repeat these five words politely after us: "Sorry, I'm too busy now."

Cry during your commute
We used to work with a woman who would get in her car after difficult days and cry her way home. By the time she pulled into her driveway, she was cleansed and had nothing to take out on family and friends. Despite how imbalanced this seems, having an emotional outlet rebalanced her.

Or try a smile
You can get angry at the unfairness of it all, or you can laugh it off, because you just can't control what others say or do, and getting angry achieves nothing. This takes practice, but in time you really can train yourself to react to the craziness of life with health-preserving zen.

Create pockets of peace

Beyond caffeine and nicotine, there's an army of everyday stimulants most people are largely unaware of. Traffic noise, background music, television, the Internet, machinery, crowds, harsh lighting... It's all stress inducing. Withstand the assault by creating (and savoring) pockets of peace in daily life. Roll up the car windows and turn off the radio. Remove televisions and computers from the bedroom. Eat more quiet dinners at home rather than at noisy restaurants. Deem one day per week information-free and don't use the Internet. Learn to cherish these oases of calm.

Drop your shoulders

Buy a pack of Post-it notes in some nice bright color. Write three words ("Drop Your Shoulders") on a dozen or so and stick them throughout your life—on your car's dashboard, inside a kitchen cabinet, on the computer monitor... Most of us live with our shoulders up around our ears, which causes headaches and neck pain. These little reminders will end that bad habit and have an amazing calming effect. The same trick works if you channel your angst in other physical habits, be it slouching, biting your nails, or playing with your hair.

Do savasana anytime

Yoga classes traditionally end with a period of relaxation called savasana. You lie on your back, close your eyes, clear your mind, and dip into the first stages of restorative sleep. Although it only lasts a few minutes, it feels delicious. But it doesn't have to be done in the context of yoga. Just close the office door or lie down on your living-room rug any time you feel like it, reminding yourself that you're not a human *doing*, you're a human *being*.

NERVES OF SEAL One of the first things Navy SEALs, military pilots, and bomb techs master is how to remain calm under pressure. No surprise there. But what is surprising is the remarkably simple way they learn this. Lieutenant Colonel David Grossman, who trains them all, begins with a lesson in breathing. The more excited or stressed you are, he explains, the quicker and shallower your respiration and the higher your blood pressure and heart rate. Most people live in this state of alert 24/7, which compromises physical and mental performance, in addition to health.

To begin changing how you breathe, do this: Put your hand on your belly and breathe normally. You'll probably notice that very little is happening down there. Now try letting your belly expand like a balloon as you inhale slowly through your nose, then let it deflate as you exhale. That's how you should be breathing all the time. The additional oxygen will nourish every cell in your body and ease your stress.

Flatten your stomach

No health book would be complete without this promise. If you believe the magazines and infomercials, this is the key to success and (of course) incredible sex. But let's be realistic. Given the cruel fact that the only time most of us will ever sport a six-pack is when we're carrying one home from the store, a different strategy is in order. Forget about crunches. Resist the urge to order the latest miracle machine by calling the toll-free number on your screen. Instead, start whittling away your middle this way.

Assess the job
Wrap a tape measure snugly around your waist, just above the hipbones. According to the Mayo Clinic, anything over 35 inches for women and 40 inches for men, regardless of your height, deserves your immediate attention.

Get the right motivation
From a health perspective belly fat is the worse kind to be saddled with. Because it's visceral (meaning it surrounds internal organs), it can increase your risk for heart disease, stroke, diabetes, and cancer. So flattening your tummy isn't solely an exercise in vanity; it's about health and living longer. And you don't have to get cover-model abs to enjoy the benefits. (There, pressure's off.)

Remember, "First to arrive, last to leave"
Fat is the ultimate bad guest. The first place it gets deposited, which is usually around the waist, is the last place it exits. So despite what the magazine covers say, you're not going to lose your gut in seven days. Try taking the long view instead: more like seven *months*.

Forget about spot reduction

It's impossible to turn fat into muscle. You could do a million sit-ups, but all that will do is make the ab muscles lying beneath your belly fat stronger. You lose belly fat by losing weight. And the best exercises for that are ones that burn the most calories, namely, aerobic activities that work the entire body.

Pull everybody's eyes up

An ornate belt or buckle, or bangles when your arms are at your sides, draw attention to your middle. Instead, wear a nice necklace, earrings, or a sporty tie, or bright shirt to keep the focus up.

Wear something naughty underneath

Slimming undergarments have come a long way since girdles and corsets. In fact, body-shaping compression wear is one of the fastest-growing clothing categories for women *and* men. Sassybax and Spanx are two popular brands. Go ahead, we won't tell anyone.

DRESS 10 POUNDS THINNER Since it takes time to lose a tummy, here are some additional dress-slimmer tips from fashion expert Stacy London:

▶▶ Instead of letting shirts hang down to your thighs, keep them at hip height. "It helps you look taller and leaner by maintaining a long leg line," she explains.

▶▶ As long as the belt doesn't have a flashy buckle that calls immediate attention to your middle, it's okay to wear one. Contrary to popular belief, London says that having a belt subtly cut across your middle helps shorten the torso and creates a longer, slimming leg line.

▶▶ In colder weather wear a sweater and keep your coat open. With a longer-style coat, this will create a vertical line that makes you look taller and thinner.

Save your marriage,
save your health

A mong all the things prescribed to better our health—exercise, weight loss, low-fat eating, checkups—rarely, if ever, are we advised to work on our marriages. Yet a landmark study at the University of Michigan determined that an unhappy marriage increases your chance of getting sick by 35 percent and shortens your life by four years. Researchers even found that happily married men and women have more white blood cells and natural killer cells in their bodies, which boosts immunity. Hmmm. Maybe it's time to take some new vows.

Exercise less

This is the only time you'll ever hear us advocate this, but marriage researcher John Gottman, PhD, makes sense when he says, "If fitness buffs spent just 10 percent of their weekly workout time—say, 20 minutes a day—working on their marriage instead of their bodies, they would get three times the health benefits." Think of it as *marital* fitness.

Kiss hello, kiss good-bye

Parting with a kiss in the morning and greeting each other with a kiss in the evening is one of the simplest ways for couples to stay connected on a daily basis. Think you're too old for that routine to make sparks fly? Rub your stocking feet on the carpet just prior to puckering up and a tiny bit of static electricity will leap from lip to lip. Yeah, you still got it.

Stop keeping score

With all due respect to Father O'Malley or Rabbi Schwartz, marriage is not a 50/50 proposition. If you're keeping tabs on whether your spouse shined the rims after you waxed the car, then, says Dr. Gottman, "you're probably not in love anymore."

Don't withdraw in a fight

Giving your spouse the silent treatment after a disagreement can be just as toxic to a relationship as yelling or calling each other names in a knock-down, drag-out battle royale, researchers have found. "Successful couples know how to exit an argument," says Dr. Gottman. Strategies include making a caring remark, offering signs of appreciation for your spouse, or simply agreeing this is "our" problem.

Teach your dog a new trick

Humor and distraction are also great ways to defuse an argument.

100 beats per minute

>> The heart rate at which arguing couples begin having trouble processing what their partner is saying.

Here's a novel idea that supplies both: Think of the phrases you and your spouse typically use during a fight. Then start repeating these whenever you play ball with your dog. In time ol' Roscoe (that's the dog, not your spouse) will recognize these "commands," grab the ball, and hopefully defuse the disagreement. Don't scoff; this is a *lot* cheaper than therapy.

Pour more of these
healthful drinks

Soda, bad. Fruit punch, bad. Sweetened teas, bad. Beer, *very* bad. Talk to someone who's serious about health and they'll tell you that many popular drinks are bad for you and that you should live mostly on ice water and hot tea. Don't take them seriously, either. There are lots of drinks that are perfectly fine for you, such as . . .

Sparkling fruit juice

One hundred percent juices, such as pome-granate, blueberry, concord grape, acai, orange, and black cherry are full of disease-fighting nutri-ents. But they're also high in calories from natural sugars and can prompt weight gain if enjoyed often. The perfect compromise? Mix an ounce or two of juice with 12 ounces of sparkling water. It tastes like soda but is much more refreshing and healthful.

Low-sodium vegetable juice cocktail

If you have the time to juice your own vegetables, then more power to you. If not, low-sodium V8 is a good alternative, especially if you have a family history of heart disease. Marie Almon, MS, RD, nutrition director for South Beach Preventive Cardiology in Miami Beach recommends six-ounce cans of vegetable juice blends. Low-sodium V8 is a good alternative, especially if you have a family history of heart disease. One 50-calorie serving contains heart-healthy fiber, lycopene, potas-sium, and vitamins A and C, while supplying less sugar than the same amount of OJ and a not-bad 140 mg of sodium.

Infused water

You'll find this offered at fancy spas, but there's no reason why you can't indulge at home. Simply fill a small pitcher with water and add prewashed fruit (lemon, berries), herbs (mint, lemongrass), or something creative (cucumber, ginger). Let it steep in the fridge overnight. Imagine you're at Canyon Ranch.

POUR LESS

Energy drinks Brands such as Red Bull, Amp, Monster, and Rockstar provide energy in unhealthful amounts from unhealthful sources. Consider:

▸▸ **Rockstar Original** (16 ounces) = sugar equivalent (62 g) of more than five servings of Froot Loops.

▸▸ **Monster Energy** (16 ounces) = caffeine equivalent (160 mg) of nearly five 12-ounce cans of Coke.

▸▸ **Amp Energy** (16 ounces) = carbohydrate equivalent (60 g) of a Burger King Whopper, and then some.

Fancy coffees A Grande drink at Starbucks is a meal in a cup. It's not surprising that America's collective rise in weight has coincided with the growth of its coffee cups.

▸▸ **Starbucks White Chocolate Mocha Frappuccino** (16 ounces with whole milk and whipped cream) = calorie equivalent (440) of a McDonald's Double Cheeseburger.

Fruit smoothie

When ordered out, this is often a health-food imposter. A 12-ounce McDonald's Wild Berry Smoothie, for example, contains about the same amount of sugar (44 g) as a can of cola.

But if you make one at home with fresh low-fat ingredients and no added sugar, it can be a nutritious and satisfying meal replacement. Combine ice, nonfat yogurt, bananas, mangoes, or whatever else fits your taste and imagination. Kids love to make them, too.

Soup

Most people don't think of soup as a drink, but it *is,* and it's extremely healthful when homemade. We always keep a carton of organic low-fat, low-sodium vegetable or chicken broth in our refrigerator. Whenever we desire a warming meal or snack, we mix some with frozen vegetables, add whole-wheat orzo or brown rice, then heat and enjoy.

Chocolate milk

Your childhood favorite can still be your adult favorite. Personal trainers actually recommend low-fat chocolate milk as a recovery drink because of the protein and other nutrients it supplies. It's also rich in calcium and vitamin D, which fights osteoporosis, and if you mix your own using unsweetened cocoa powder, there's even evidence it aids the cardiovascular system by reducing inflammation. Plus, you always looked good with a mustache.

Managing
the system

Stress is a major underlying cause of disease and death, which is why it's so ironic (and sad) that our healthcare system is dispensing so much of it. If you're often frustrated, confused, or overwhelmed by medical and dietary options, this section will show you how to gain more control and make smarter decisions. Whether you're trying to find the best doctors or vitamins, a top-notch surgeon or workout, consider this your GPS for getting where you want to go with minimal hassle.

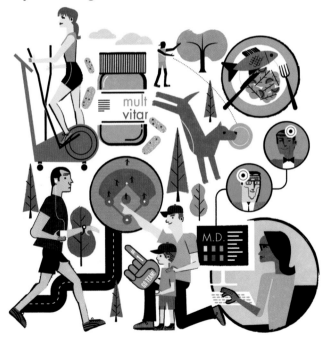

Find a
top-notch doc

The partner who has the most potential to influence your life is not the one sleeping beside you every night. Rather, it's one most people choose with far less care than the decision deserves. We're talking about your family doctor—the general practitioner or internist who is the first line in your health defense and, thus, your *real* life partner. Here's how to find one you love.

See what's possible
Given the cost of healthcare, you'll need to work within the confines of your insurance plan (assuming you have one). So begin by perusing its list of local in-network physicians. Some plans have started grading participating doctors. See if yours does.

Ask around
Friends, family, other doctors, nurses, even the health reporter at your local newspaper are all great sources for referrals. Google also has a free service, called Aardvark (vark. com), which taps your immediate and extended on-line social network to get quick answers to questions like this.

Check the record
See if the doctors you're considering are licensed to practice in your state and whether they've had any disciplinary action

(fsmb.org/directory_smb.html). Check also who's board certified (abms.org), meaning they've passed additional exams and participate in ongoing education. Then search their names on the Internet. Although you can't trust everything there, it may turn up additional insights.

Go undercover

Call the office of each doc on your shortlist and ask some basic questions, such as if they're open on evenings and weekends or use nurse practitioners or doctor's assistants. More important than the answers is how long it takes to get a real person on the line and how pleasant and efficient they seem. Then visit the office to see what kind of vibe you get.

> "Never go to a doctor whose office plants have died."
> —Erma Bombeck

How long does it take before someone greets you? Does the staff look happy and in control? What's the mood in the waiting room? Even go as far as to take a seat, mention you are doctor shopping, and listen to patient opinions.

Look for a connection

Doctors are extremely busy, but try to chat face-to-face for a few minutes with your finalists. Does he look fit and healthy? Does she look you in the eyes and listen? Some experts recommend choosing a doctor who's the same sex and age as you because they'll supposedly better identify with the stage of life you're in.

Be persistent

If the doctor you want is not taking new patients, that's a good sign. Ask another doctor you're seeing for a referral or get on the waiting list.

Cut healthcare costs

The system is screwed up. No doubt about it. But a good deal of the blame rests with us. Because of the traditional trust placed in doctors, we rarely apply even basic consumerism to the medical profession. We've forgotten that we're *customers*—free to second-guess, shop around, negotiate, choose, and demand satisfaction. If that surprises you, it shouldn't. It's your right. Here's how to stand up, take control, and save a few bucks.

Shop at home
The best way to reduce medical costs is a step you're already taking. Educating yourself about health and implementing the lifestyle changes in this book (losing weight, exercising regularly, eating smarter, quitting bad habits...) will help you stay healthy. Prevention is the best investment.

Don't bother the gods with little things
Emergency rooms and doctors' offices are the Ritz-Carltons of healthcare venues: the most expensive locales in town. If the need isn't critical, visit an urgent-care facility or one of the new retail health clinics in supermarkets and department stores instead. (But check with your healthcare provider first to be sure you're covered there.) Many retail clinics also offer free periodic health screenings.

Negotiate everything
If you can summon the gumption to do so, you'll find there are more options (and savings) available than you ever thought possible. Here's a quick list of responses to some common scenarios:

Doctor orders...	*You politely inquire...*
▶▶ **A prescription**	*Is there a suitable generic or any free samples?*
▶▶ **A medical test**	*Where's the most affordable place to get it?*
▶▶ **Minor surgery**	*Possible at an outpatient clinic instead of the hospital?*
▶▶ **Follow-up appointment**	*Can it be done by phone or video chat?*
▶▶ **Payment**	*I can't afford this; is there anything you can do?*

Consider canceling dental and vision coverage

Compare your annual premium and copays from the previous year with the actual benefits you received. You may find it's cheaper to forgo coverage and just pay cash whenever these services are required. In fact, some dentists and optometrists will actually give you a cash discount.

Admit that times are tough

If you lose your healthcare coverage or can't afford the deductible costs or copays for medications, tests, or treatments, tell your doctor. Many physicians will discount services, offer a payment plan, or at least direct you to clinics or programs for people in need.

If all else fails, try bartering

If you happen to be an electrician or plumber, you may never have to pay for healthcare again.

Best **20** minute workout:
Interval training

To get the most benefit from limited exercise time, do interval training, says Arthur Agastson, the heart doctor who founded the South Beach Diet. This involves systematically raising and lowering your heart rate over the course of a workout. Doing so has many benefits: Interval training strengthens the cardiovascular system, burns additional calories and fat, combats boredom, boosts fitness, and lowers insulin levels/resistance. Plus, the concept can be applied to just about any activity, from walking or biking to using indoor machines like stationary bikes and elliptical trainers. Here's a simple schedule you can follow (once you're cleared by your doctor). There's no need for a heart-rate monitor, just base your pace on "perceived exertion" or how you feel.

1. *Warm up for 3 minutes at a comfortable pace.*

2. *Do six 30-second intervals, alternating 15 seconds at a faster pace with 15 seconds at normal pace.*

3. *Do eight 60-second intervals, alternating 30 seconds at a faster pace with 30 seconds at normal pace.*

4. *Do six 30-second intervals, alternating 15 seconds at a faster pace with 15 seconds at normal pace.*

5. *Cool down for 3 minutes at a comfortable pace.*

6. *Do this workout every other day, adjusting the number and length of the intervals as your fitness improves.*

PERSONAL N●TES

{ How can I get **more movement** into my day? }

Make sense
of media health reports

Ope day eggs are bad for you; the next day they're beneficial. One day vitamin E supplements are great for the
heart; the next day they're not. On one visit your doctor tells
you to boost good cholesterol, but on another he's not even
sure it's "good" anymore. And the list goes on. It seems that
practically every week there's another news report about a
study contradicting some aspect of healthful living previously
considered gospel. If you're increasingly frustrated and confused by such flip-flops, a little perspective can go a long way.

Don't immediately swallow it

Despite being performed by MDs and PhDs, health studies
are often initially interpreted by reporters with far less expertise. Plus, the unfortunate inclination of today's media is to
sensationalize things, especially on news crawls and websites,
where boosting page views and beating the competition are
paramount. So don't practice knee-jerk medicine by starting (or
stopping) anything based on a first report.

Study the study

ScienceDaily.com provides accurate and balanced study sum-
maries, plus links to the source of the story. Bookmark it. To have
merit, a study must meet certain criteria: It should be conducted
by a reputable person or organization (the National Institutes
of Health or the Cleveland Clinic, for instance). It should be (or
about to be) published in a respected, peer-reviewed journal (i.e.,
the *New England Journal of Medicine*). It should use a fairly
large sample (thousands rather than dozens) of humans (not lab
animals). And it should be independent (free of influence from

sponsors with vested interests). If any of these conditions are not met, be suspect.

Wait for reaction

Single studies rarely change medicine. In the weeks following the initial report, doctors and other experts will interpret the findings and put them in context with other research. Unfortunately, this perspective is not usually reported at the same fever pitch, if at all. So wait a week or two and then Google "reaction/implications to XXX study" to determine what to do.

Accept that science is fluid

As technology advances, it allows us to examine things in new ways. Pluto, for example, is no longer a planet, and we now know that bacteria rather than stress cause ulcers. So don't view shifting science as evidence of disarray and allow it to demoralize you. Instead, welcome it as refinement and, with the help of your doctor, apply it.

SO IS IT GOOD OR BAD?

▶▶ **Butter:** High in cholesterol and saturated fat. Minimize.

▶▶ **Margarine:** Trans fat–free tubs or liquids are a better choice than butter.

▶▶ **Eggs:** No more than four yolks per week, if you're cholesterol sensitive.

▶▶ **Coffee:** One or two cups per day of regular are fine, but decaf is best.

▶▶ **Beef:** Okay if it's lean and the serving size is 3 to 6 ounces.

Buy the best
vitamins

How big is the health supplements industry? Let's put it this way: Americans spend as much on vitamins in a year as they do on movie tickets (just over $10 billion for each). No doubt, your kitchen or medicine cabinet is lined with vitamin bottles. Yet this vast market is largely unregulated. The government does not verify a product's ingredients, claims, or even safety before it goes on sale. Plus, recent studies have raised doubts about the effectiveness of such bestsellers as multivitamins, antioxidants, and even vitamin C. To be sure you're taking quality products that will improve rather than hurt your health, here's what to do.

Think big picture

Vitamins and supplements may not be medicine, but they're still pills that introduce chemicals into your body. And that means they can interact with one another and prescription medications. For instance, if you're taking calcium to prevent osteoporosis, are you aware it could reduce the effectiveness of some antibiotics? Likewise, fish oil can interfere with some blood-pressure drugs. So everything you're taking must be viewed in concert. The National Institutes of Health's website medlineplus.gov lists the efficacy, safety concerns, and side effects of 100 popular herbs and supplements. Use this information and the advice of your doctor to decide what (if anything) you should take.

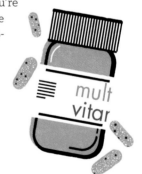

Find a reputable brand

Even if a particular vitamin or herb has a good deal of supporting research, this doesn't mean the brand you're buying contains a high grade of it. This is where an organization called U.S. Pharmacopeia (usp.org) comes in. It independently verifies the quality, purity, and potency of dietary supplements and their ingredients. Look for the USP VERIFIED insignia on labels and/or visit the USP website to check individual products. Note that USP only examines products that manufacturers voluntarily submit, so it's not comprehensive.

VITAMIN BS

One-Third »The amount of supplements analyzed by consumer groups that contained doses much lower or higher than stated on their labels.

Do the vinegar test

We have a friend who once had a CT scan that showed a blotch in her lower intestine. She was relieved but surprised to learn it was an undigested multivitamin. To be sure your supplements are dissolving inside you as they're supposed to, drop one of each in a glass of vinegar. If they're still there thirty minutes later, then they're just commuting through your small intestine, where most nutrients are absorbed, and you should try another brand.

Get what you need from food

When it comes to supplements, there may very well be no magic pill. Scientists are finding that when micronutrients like antioxidants are isolated and taken on their own, they don't have the same health benefits as when they're consumed naturally in food. So the smartest plan of all may be what you've known all along: Eat as varied a diet as possible of whole foods, fresh fruit, and vegetables.

Outsmart
a restaurant menu

Seventy-one percent of adults say they're trying to eat more healthfully at restaurants, according to a recent poll. But good intention and resisting temptation are two entirely different things. For proof, look around the next time you're at one of those Chinese buffets and see how many people are loading up on steamed bean curd. If you travel a lot for business or eat out frequently with family and friends, here's how to stick to your guns and finally tighten those buns.

Take home half of what you order
If you're at a restaurant that's renowned for its large portions, like The Cheesecake Factory, tell the waitress to put half your meal in a doggie bag *before* she brings it to the table. This will ensure you don't overeat, and you'll end up with a ready-made lunch for the next day.

Create your own Special of the Day
A menu is really just an organized inventory of what's in the kitchen. You're free to have those ingredients prepared or paired any way you like. So order the fish grilled with lemon rather than broiled in butter, swap the creamy coleslaw for a side salad, and ask for a baked potato rather than French fries—in other words, *you* be the chef.

Use these tricks at the trough
All-you-can-eat restaurants are generally the least healthful dining-out option. But if you find yourself at one, try to sit at a booth rather than a table and face away from the buffet. Make sure to browse the food first; otherwise, you'll just keep piling

food on your plate as you encounter items you like. Also choose the smallest serving plate available. And when it's finally time to chow, put a napkin on your lap (for some reason, it makes you less likely to keep getting up for more). Researchers have found that doing all these things significantly reduces the amount of food you eat.

Make a meal of appetizers
These are usually smaller portions, and there are a lot to choose from on most menus. So make believe you're at a Spanish tapas restaurant and order two or three as your main meal.

Have less room for macaroons
If dessert is your downfall, always order a cup of healthy soup (vegetable, noodle, tomato) or a slice of bread with two table-spoons of dipping olive oil as your starter. Either option will fill you up so you'll eat less later. In fact, olive oil prompts the release of a stomach hormone called cholecystokinin, which suppresses appetite.

NEVER ORDER THIS

▸▸ **Chef Salad:** With dressing, it's about 1,400 calories.

▸▸ **Prime Rib:** A typical cut has as many calories and as much fat as a Big Mac.

▸▸ **Caesar Salad:** Can be up to 80 percent fat because of all the oil and cheese it's pre-tossed with.

▸▸ **Nachos:** Melted cheese on top of fatty beef on top of fried chips. A few chopped tomatoes and onions can't rescue that.

▸▸ **Pizza with the works:** Sausage, pepperoni and salami are among the fattiest meats on the planet.

Wait less
in waiting rooms

One of the underlying reasons many people don't take better care of themselves is because the process of seeing a doctor can be interminable. You have to jockey for an appointment weeks in advance, take time off from work, then sit (and sit) in a room surrounded by patients (and old magazines) you hope aren't contagious. Here are the best ways we've found to spend far less time waiting in waiting rooms.

Schedule a virtual house call
Ask the office if your doctor does web conferencing or videophone consults. If so and you have the right equipment (computer/webcam/Internet or 3G/4G videophone), he'll be able to answer your questions, review reports, and even conduct limited physical exams without you needing to go anywhere.

Book these slots
If a face-to-face is necessary, reserve the first or second appointment of the day to minimize the risk of being delayed. The first slot after lunch is also good (if the doctor breaks for one). Bonus: You may even get better care because the staff is fresher.

Have your paperwork ready
When making your appointment, ask if any extensive forms have to be filled out. If so, either pick them up or have them faxed or mailed to you so you can complete them beforehand.

Health... The Reader's Digest VERSION

Call ahead

If you have an appointment later in the day, call the office an hour before leaving to see if the doctor is on schedule. If not, delay your arrival accordingly. At the very least, you'll indicate to the receptionist that you're a busy person, which might get you more timely attention. For an ER visit that doesn't involve a life-threatening situation, call ahead as well or go in the early morning, when it's usually calmer.

Take emergency measures

OK, this strategy can only ever be used once, but if you really need to get in and out of a doctor's office fast, tell the receptionist a family or work emergency has come up and request to be the next patient seen. For ER visits ask your doctor to call ahead and notify the staff you're coming in. This may give you higher priority.

Visit the supermarket

For minor infections, immunizations, and routine health screenings, visit one of the independent medical clinics that have opened recently in drugstores, supermarkets, and even Walmart. They're usually staffed by physicians or certified nurse practitioners, have convenient hours, and charge less than traditional docs. But what's most attractive is that no appointment is necessary. Even if there's a line, you can grab a call buzzer and shop while you wait.

DON'T MIND WAITING Instead of stressing out about waiting, treat it as an opportunity to relax—some precious downtime in your demanding day. Start the novel you've been anxious to read, watch a movie on your laptop, listen to a lecture from ted. com on your mobile or iPod, or just close your eyes and take a nap. It isn't a disruption; it's a gift.

Make these health moves in
your 30s

What	When
Routine checks/exams	
Complete physical	Every 5 years
Blood pressure	Every 6 months
Cholesterol	Every 5 years
Blood glucose	Every 3 years
Eyesight	Every 5 years
Teeth	Twice yearly
Hearing	At least once this decade
Body mass index (BMI)	Every 6 months
Skin cancer	Every 3 years
Testicular cancer	Monthly self-exam
Mammogram	Periodically *(if at risk; ask your doctor)*
Pelvic exam/Pap test	Every 2 to 3 years
Thyroid	Every 5 years > age 35

Health... The Reader's Digest VERSION

This go-go decade of career- and family-building is when many root causes of disease gain a foothold. These include chronic stress, inadequate sleep, poor nutrition, and weight gain. While it's not easy to find time for yourself amidst everything else, the less you let slip away now the less you'll have to make up later.

Inoculations

Influenza	Annually
Tetanus-diphtheria	Once per decade
Others	If missed in prior decade (see page 42)

General

Find a life partner.	Married people live longer.
Manage stress.	Nothing is more debilitating long term.
Prioritize sleep.	Adults need 8 to 9 hours nightly...*really.*
Eat smart to control weight.	Metabolism is on the decline.
Enjoy your endurance.	It peaks during this decade.

Negotiate
an emergency room

Four hours and seven minutes. That's the average wait time you can expect in a hospital emergency room. To put this in perspective, that's just enough time to watch the entire *Kill Bill* box set or almost as long as Britney Spears and Jason Alexander were married. Here's how to get in and out of an ER with the care you need much more efficiently.

Head to another state (if you live in Utah)
ER patients there wait the longest of anywhere—an average of 8 hours, 17 minutes.

Do your homework
Not all surgery or trauma centers are accredited, so find out which ones in your area are, before an emergency happens. Do this by 1) checking for accreditation by the American College of Surgeons (facs.org/trauma), 2) determining how close you are to a top-rated Level I or II trauma facility (cdc.gov/traumacare), and 3) asking doctors, nurses, friends, and even local EMT crew for their opinions about the best emergency care in your region.

Make sure you're in the right place
The reason wait times are so long is because ERs are overwhelmed (often, the delay is finding beds in a hospital for admitted patients). If there's a life-threatening situation (loss of consciousness, signs of heart attack or stroke, severe pain, heavy bleeding) don't hesitate in getting to one. But if it's a minor burn, bite, break, illness, or irritation, save time and money by visiting an urgent-care center. These offer a middle ground between doctors' offices and emergency rooms. If in doubt about what to do in a non–life threatening situation, contact your doctor.

Pick your time

If treatment can wait for a little while, most ERs and urgent-care centers often are least busy between 3:00 and 9:00 a.m.

Call an ambulance

If it's a serious situation, EMTs will not only start treatment but also call ahead so the hospital is prepared for your arrival. That saves critical time compared to just showing up.

Practice full disclosure

No matter how embarrassing or intimate the accident or affliction, telling the medical staff everything will get you faster, more focused care. This extends to health history, current medications, and even supplements you're taking. Consider wearing a medical ID bracelet or necklace in case you're unconscious. New models contain downloadable flash drives.

Look on the bright side

The longer you're kept waiting, the less serious your condition probably is. It's the grave situations that get treated first. Nonetheless, don't be shy about periodically checking with the nurses as to when you'll be seen, but make sure to do it politely.

MOST COMMON ER ERROR? Medication mistakes, says Bryan Bledsoe, DO, a professor of emergency medicine at the University of Nevada School of Medicine. To protect yourself amidst all the commotion, get the nurse or doctor to do a double check by asking what the medication is, who it's for, and why you're getting it. Dr. Bledsoe says these three simple questions will prevent most errors.

Buy generic
or brand drugs

GENERIC

When your doctor prescribes a generic drug, you usually don't think twice about it. After all, it's cheaper than the marquee version, your insurance company won't object, plus it's the same thing, right? Well, not exactly. Here's how to make sure your generic doesn't cause any hysterics.

Understand the difference
After the patent on a brand drug expires, other companies can produce copies and, because they incurred none of the R&D costs, sell them for less. By law the active ingredients and dosages must remain the same, but the inactive ones (fillers, colors, flavorings, preservatives) can change. The FDA allows generic drugs to have a blood serum level of 80 to 125 percent of the blood serum level produced by ingesting the brand-name product. Therefore, generics are similar (or "bioequivalent," as the FDA terms it) but not clones. As a result, there have been some reports of varying levels of potency and effectiveness.

Keep things in perspective
Seventy percent of all the prescriptions filled in the United States are for generics, saving consumers 80 to 85 percent, or $8 to $10 billion annually. That's a tremendous benefit. And the vast majority of people encounter no safety or efficacy issues. Nonetheless . . .

Don't give in to pressure
If your healthcare provider or doctor wants you to switch to a generic, be sure it's in your best interest. Watchdog groups such as the National Consumers League point out that insurers are out to reduce costs, and some doctors receive incentives from

pharmaceutical reps. There are some drug categories, notably antidepressants, proton-pump inhibitors, and epileptic and cardiovascular medications that may be less well suited for generic substitution. If you're feeling strong-armed, get a second opinion from another doctor or pharmacist or file an appeal with your insurance provider.

Don't switch on your own

In most cases pharmacies will allow you to swap a generic for a brand prescription, but don't make that snap decision without first consulting your doctor. Some meds, such as blood thinners and thyroid drugs, have a "narrow therapeutic index." This means the margin of safety between benefit and risk is relatively small and any substitution must be closely monitored, if permitted at all.

Become more self-aware

If you switch to a generic after successfully taking a brand drug for a while, report any changes you experience to your doctor. If you're taking statins to manage cholesterol, schedule a blood test sooner than usual to compare the generic's effectiveness. Likewise, if you opt for a generic hypertension med, take your blood pressure more often in the ensuing weeks. Keep in mind that pharmacies can source generics from different manufacturers, so always compare labels when picking up a new batch.

THE BEST OF BOTH WORLDS? In the near future you may have a third option beyond just generic and brand-name drugs. Pharmaceutical giants such as Eli Lilly, Pfizer, and Abbott Labs are getting into the generic-drug business with so-called "branded generics." These medications are an appealing compromise for many who desire a trusted brand at a more affordable price. Although primarily being marketed in Europe and Asia at the moment, they could gain a bigger foothold here.

Assess
alternative therapies

In a classic case of "the grass is always greener," Western consumers are turning toward Eastern and alternative health remedies (38 percent of Americans spending $34 billion annually), while our counterparts around the world continue viewing the United States as the medical leader. Who's right? Probably both, but until the two schools merge, here's how to weigh your options.

Remember these two important things

Manufacturers of dietary supplements do not have to prove the safety or efficacy of their products before selling them (and "natural" doesn't mean "safe"). There is also no standardized national system for credentialing complementary and alternative medicine (CAM) practitioners. So this is largely a Wild West market, and you need to be a wary hombre.

But there is a government agency...

It's called the National Center for Complementary and Alternative Medicine. It's a clearinghouse for education and research, and its excellent website (nccam.nih.gov) should be your first stop when considering any unconventional treatment. It offers background on specific therapies, a link to the FDA's Health Fraud Awareness page, and even information specialists who can help with research.

Watch for red-flag words

Miracle cure, revolutionary discovery, secret ingredient, ancient remedy, cure-all, purify, detoxify, energize...These are all descriptions designed to excite rather than inform. When you see any of them on a website or advertisement, beware. It's even worse if "operators are standing by to take your order on this special one-time offer."

Consider the cost

Although some healthcare plans cover chiropractic, acupuncture, and massage, most CAM therapies must be paid for out of pocket. And some are pretty expensive. Ask your provider about the extent of your policy before scheduling treatment.

Let your doctor be your guide

Even though general practitioners are conventionally trained, most are familiar with alternative therapies and can help assess the relative risks and benefits (and maybe even the practitioner or manufacturer). More important, your doctor will warn you if a supplement could interact with what you're already taking. For instance, taking ginkgo biloba if you're already on Coumadin could raise your risk of internal bleeding, since both are blood thinners.

Consider integrating

If you're dissatisfied with your doctor or current mode of treatment but still want to explore CAM therapies with a safety net, consider integrative medicine. It combines conventional with complementary therapies in a best-of-both-world's approach. Check with the most respected medical facility in your area to see if it does.

YOU: A GUINEA PIG One way to be on the cusp of alternative healthcare is to participate in a clinical trial. These are research studies in which specific therapies are evaluated. The National Center for Complementary and Alternative Medicine maintains a database of trials where you can see what's upcoming and how you can register. Although there are risks involved (after all, these treatments are experimental), depending on where you're at in the management of your condition, it might be worthwhile. For more information, visit nccam.nih.gov/research/clinicaltrials/factsheet.

Buy medicine
online safely

Online shopping is fun, convenient, and economical, but buying pills on the Internet is a lot different than purchasing a jacket from landsend.com. To date the National Association of Boards of Pharmacy (NABP) has reviewed more than 8,000 online-pharmacy websites and only 4 percent "appear to be in compliance with pharmacy laws and practice standards." This means if you're not careful about buying drugs online, the health of you and your family could be in jeopardy.

Click off the "no prescription necessary" sites
No matter how tempting it may be to order drugs such as Viagra without the embarrassment of seeing a doctor, if an online seller doesn't require a prescription, there's a good chance the pills you receive (if you get them at all) will be counterfeit, improperly formulated, or expired.

Check the hit list
The NABP publishes lists of "recommended" and "not recommended" online pharmacies at nabp.net. Or just look for the blue-and-red VIPPS seal on the pharmacy's home page. It stands for Verified Internet Pharmacy Practices Sites and signifies compliance with NABP standards and state and federal laws. (Your healthcare provider may also be able to recommend reputable online services.)

Beware of those Canadians
Although there are legitimate Canadian online pharmacies with attractive prices, the FDA prohibits foreign countries from selling prescription drugs to Americans, because it can't ensure the

safety and efficacy of those products. So despite how trustworthy these sites appear to be, when they try to tap the American market, they're operating illegally.

Compare prices

Don't assume you always get the best deal online. With the advent of pharmacies at Walmart and Target, along with the proliferation of generics, by the time you pay for shipping and handling or overnight delivery, your savings may not be that substantial. In fact, it may pay you to develop a relationship with a local pharmacist, who you can use as a resource. For price comparisons at NABP-accredited online pharmacies, use the search engine at pharmahelper.com.

Watch the weather forecast

Drugs can lose their potency in extreme conditions (which is why they shouldn't be stored in a hot, steamy bathroom). In fact, researchers in Phoenix found that the asthma medication formoterol significantly degraded after as little as 30 minutes at 158°F (70°C)—a common temperature in sealed metal mailboxes or delivery trucks in that part of the country. Check if your meds have temperature recommendations on their labels. If so, either ask your online supplier to ship accordingly or buy locally.

PILLS FOR PETS If you have pets, you know how expensive keeping them healthy can get. And ordering medications over the Internet carries the same risks for them as it does for you. The National Association Boards of Pharmacy also accredits online pharmacies that sell prescription drugs for animals. Look for the brown "Vet-VIPPS" symbol on the site's home page or visit nabp.net for a complete list of accredited businesses.

Find a
stellar surgeon

You don't take your car to just any mechanic to get it repaired; you ask around first. Same with finding someone to remodel your kitchen, landscape your yard, or do your income tax. So why are people so trusting when it comes to hospitals and surgeons? They shouldn't be. Primary-care doctors often belong to broad groups of medical practitioners. For financial reasons some refer to specialists within their group, even though they may not be the most qualified. No wonder that since 1999 an estimated 1 million people have died and countless more have been injured by faulty medical care. In fact, according to the Institute of Medicine, medical error is the eighth leading cause of death in the United States. Here's how to protect yourself and your loved ones.

Examine the doctor

Visit absurgery.org to see if your surgeon is certified by the American Board of Surgery. If yes, ask him two key questions. First, is he current on all training requirements, especially as it pertains to the procedure you're about to undergo? As with all professions, methods and standards change constantly in medicine, and doctors need to stay up to date. Then ask how many surgeries like yours he's performed. "Healthcare is like sports," says the director of a major training hospital. "The more you practice, the better you become." (See also "Find a Top-Notch Doc," page 62.)

Ask if he plays Nintendo

No kidding. Studies have shown that video gaming systems such as Nintendo Wii (and the game Marble Mania, in particular) hone the same motor and perception skills used in laparoscopic surgery. In fact, surgeons at Banner Simulation Medical Center in Arizona, who train on the Wii, make fewer errors.

Chat with the nurses

Visit the hospital floor where the surgery will be done and ask the nurses this question: "If you or a family member were having this operation, which doctor would you choose?" They'll give you an unbiased opinion. Or speak with the hospital's pathologists. They perform autopsies and witness firsthand the results of operations.

> "It is a mathematical fact that 50 percent of all doctors graduate in the bottom half of their class."
>
> —Anonymous

Check the hospital's infection rate

If the procedure will involve insertion of a central venous catheter, ask your doctor for the hospital's rate of central-line infection. If it's more than 3 in 100 (or the doctor doesn't know), look elsewhere.

Write on yourself

Although it sounds unbelievable, it's smart to write "cut here" or "this knee" on your skin with a permanent marker. And up until you drift off, ask every hospital employee you meet, "What operation am I having done?" Better safe than scheduled for follow-up surgery.

Shop like a
nutritionist

Imagine if you were able to look over the shoulder of a mechanic diagnosing car trouble or assist a master chef preparing dinner for six. You'd learn a ton because experts like these know all the tricks. So we decided to shadow some nutritionists on a trip to the supermarket. Here are their secrets for getting in, getting out, and most important, getting you healthy.

Eat something beforehand

Shopping on an empty stomach is like walking the dog past a Krispy Kreme donut shop. No matter how pure your intentions, you'll undoubtedly glaze over and succumb to temptation. Nutritionists always shop after—never before—meals.

Come with a plan

The experts never wing it. They devise a healthful meal plan ahead of time and make a list of all the necessary ingredients. This keeps them focused.

Hire a surrogate shopper

Believe it or not, some nutritionists don't shop. Instead, they e-mail their list to the supermarket and have their order delivered. Although this costs extra, they find it actually saves money (and time) because they don't buy items on impulse. Alternatively, one nutritionist has her husband or son do the shopping. This strategy is based on a Food Marketing Institute survey that concluded guys are more likely than women to stick to a grocery list. (Warning: This approach does not work with men at Home Depot.)

Grab a smaller cart

This trick employs the same psychology as eating from smaller dinner plates or bowls when you're trying to lose weight. With limited space you won't overbuy and, later, overeat.

Patrol the perimeter first

Traditionally, the outer supermarket aisles are where the freshest, most healthful foods are located—meats, fish, fruits, dairy, vegetables . . . Nutritionists make the bulk of their buys here.

Make quick turns and look up and down

When they must delve into the middle of the store, nutritionists usually ignore the displays at the heads of the aisles and most everything at eye level. This is where you typically find chips, cookies, soda, and other less nutritious (but highly profitable) items.

WANT NOT, WASTE NOT

12 » Percent of a typical grocery order that people don't eat and eventually throw away.

Look for short ingredient lists

To keep from getting bogged down reading labels, nutritionists often buy the brand with the fewest ingredients. These are generally the least processed and thus are more natural and better for you. (For more label-reading tips, see page 22.)

Shadow your own nutritionist

Some supermarket chains employ regional nutritionists to lead customer-education efforts. If you make a reservation in advance, some will even act as your personal shopper, accompanying you through the store and helping to amend your diet.

Know when to
see a doctor

Most guys would rather tough it out, women are often too busy, and the dog and cat generally prefer to just lick it. Sometimes, though, seeing a doctor is what you need to do, and pronto. Here's how to know when you've crossed that line.

» Ankle injury
Pain and swelling doesn't subside after a few days.

» Backache
Persistent and disabling.

» Bleeding
Any blood coming from any place you've never seen it before.

» Bug bite
Bull's-eye-type rash with a red center and ring, accompanied by flulike symptoms and joint pain, especially if you live in an area where Lyme disease is prevalent.

» Chest discomfort
Pressure or pain in the middle of the chest, with shortness of breath, nausea, cold sweats, or tingling in the arms.

» Cold
Persists more than 10 days or is accompanied by high fever, significantly swollen glands, or severe sinus pain.

» Constipation
Lasts more than two weeks and is generally unresponsive to laxatives or is accompanied by intense abdominal/rectal pain.

» Cough
Produces pinkish or greenish yellow phlegm, plus difficulty breathing and fever.

» Earache
Persists more than a day, with pain and discharge.

» Fever
Lasts more than three days or is higher than 103°F (39°C).

» Headache
Sudden, severe, or accompanied by confusion, fainting, dizziness, slurred speech, blurred vision, nausea, high fever, or numbness.

» Lumps
Anything that pops up anywhere without an identifiable cause, whether it hurts or not.

» Nausea
Vomiting lasts more than two days, inability to drink for 24 hours, history of heart disease or diabetes.

» Peeing
If the urge becomes frequent, the process is painful, or if the urine has a reddish tinge not attributable to diet or medication.

» Postpartum sadness
Baby blues lasting longer than two weeks and accompanied by withdrawal, mood swings, or thoughts of harming the infant.

» Pain
Anything unusual, severe, or stubborn.

» Snoring
Regularly waking up with a choking snort that leaves you breathless, plus excessive daytime drowsiness.

» Sore throat

Unusually severe, lasting longer than a week, or is joined by fever, difficulty breathing, or blood-tinged saliva.

» Spots

Any noticeable change to the shape, color, or size of a mole, freckle, or other patch of skin.

» Stress

When it results in a significant decline of work/school performance, excess anxiety, misuse of alcohol/drugs, irrational fears, changes in sleeping/eating habits, sustained withdrawal, or suicidal thoughts.

» Weight loss

Any significant drop not resulting from a change in diet, exercise, or illness.

GET IN LINE

10 ⁇ Percent of office visits that physicians say could have been "self-managed" by the patient.

52.6 million ⁇ Number of office visits that 10 percent figure equates to.

$10.4 billion ⁇ Amount of money all those unnecessary visits cost consumers and taxpayers.

Source: 2008 Consumer Healthcare Products Association survey

Best (30) minute workout:
Run/walk

Nothing beats running for a quick, thorough, cardiovascular workout. Plus, it burns lots of calories, tones leg muscles, and is so simple and convenient it can be done anywhere. But if you're out of shape or new to running, you don't want to lace on your shoes and take off for a half hour. That'll be too exhausting, and you could injure yourself in the process. Instead, after checking with your doctor, taper into the activity by following this 30-minute program from the folks at *Runner's World* magazine. In just seven short weeks you'll be running the entire time, and a whole new world of health and fitness will open up.

▸▸ *The Code*
W = Walk	m = minutes
R = Run	x = times (as in repeat 6x)

▸▸ *The Frequency*
Do each workout four times per week (i.e., Monday, Wednesday, Friday, and Saturday). On other days either walk for 30 minutes (Tuesday and Thursday) or rest entirely (Sunday). As far as pace, maintain what's comfortably challenging.

▸▸ *The Plan*

Week 1: Walk for 30 minutes

Week 2: 4mW/1mR, 6x = (6 total minutes of running)

Week 3: 2mW/1mR, 10x = (10 total minutes of running)

Week 4: 1mR/1mW, 15x = (15 total minutes of running)

Week 5: 2mR/1mW, 10x = (20 total minutes of running)

Week 6: 4mR/1mW, 6x = (24 total minutes of running)

Week 7: Run for 30 minutes

Find the right diet for you

Search "diet books" on Amazon and you'll find 56,513 options. Eat baby food to lose weight! Oops, didn't work? Try these doctor-endorsed cookies instead! No, no, the answer is caveman cuisine! Wait, our mistake. Listen to Marie Osmond, Kirstie Alley, or Alicia Silverstone....If you're confused, overwhelmed, or if it feels like you've personally tried every one of these 56,513 plans and still don't have the body you want, it's time to regroup.

Get your terms straight

One of the reasons this country is so fat is because most people don't understand the meaning of the word "diet."

POPULAR DEFINITION	PROPER DEFINITION
Short term	Long term
Fad	Lifestyle
Celebrity	Reality
Elimination	Moderation
Losing weight	Staying healthy

See the difference? A diet shouldn't be a fast fix; it should be a life plan. To tell one from the other is a simple matter of asking, Can I eat this way for the rest of my life? If the answer is no, don't even try it.

Simplify the science

A study reported in the *New England Journal of Medicine* tracked 811 overweight adults on a variety of low-carb, low-fat, high-protein diets. Most of the diets had fancy theories and narrow research findings behind them that, when read in isolation, sounded awfully convincing. Several were detailed in bestselling books. And yet, after two years no single diet emerged as the best. "The real key," says J. Graham Thomas, PhD, at the

Weight Control and Diabetes Research Center in Rhode Island, "is energy balance. To lose weight you must burn more energy than you eat, and for weight maintenance the two must be in balance." You don't need a magic diet to accomplish this; you just need the knowledge and resolve to ensure that activity cancels out calories every day.

Understand your daily cycle

So how do you begin to get a handle on daily energy balance? One convenient tool that's worked for many people is a mobile phone app called Lose It! It's a daily calorie and exercise tracker that you can download for free from your favorite app store (or visit loseit.com to learn more). Using it over time imparts a better sense of how nutrition and activity work together. Indeed, in an ongoing study of 6,000 people who have lost at least 30 pounds and kept it off for a year or more, a key to success is daily self-monitoring just like that. "These people know on a daily basis whether they're heading in the right direction or not," explains Thomas. Tracking food intake, weight, and physical activity lets them make instant adjustments.

HOW FAD DIETS MAKE YOU FAT Your body can't tell the difference between dieting and starving. Any time you significantly cut calories for an extended period, your body automatically lowers its metabolism to conserve energy and protect its existence. But when you can no longer endure the crazy diet you're on and food reappears, metabolism stays low and the additional calories are stored as fat in anticipation of the next "famine."

Although it's a remarkably efficient system for ensuring the continuation of the species, it condemns those who repeatedly experience it to even higher weights and body-fat percentages. This is the curse of "weight cycling" or "yo-yo dieting." To avoid it, make sure any weight-loss program you embark on is slow, sustainable, and accompanied by exercise.

Stay calm in an MRI

Some medical sounds scare the bejeebers out of us. There's the high-pitched whir of a dentist's drill, the flat-line whine of an EKG, and perhaps worst of all, that incessant banging during an MRI. While there's not much you can do about the first two, there are plenty of ways to make an MRI more bearable.

Understand what's happening

As with anything, the more information you have, the less anxious you'll be. (And about 15 percent of MRI patients become too nervous to proceed.) MRI stands for Magnetic Resonance Imaging. As you remain motionless in the scanner, radio waves in a magnetic field produce detailed images of your insides. The process is safer and more precise than X-rays, and that banging noise is the normal sound of the scanner's gradient coils and magnetic fields at work.

Ask about an open MRI

Because of their tunnel-like design, traditional closed scanners can trigger claustrophobia and panic attacks. Newer, open scanners aren't as confining and reduce those risks. But not all facilities have them, and depending on what you're getting done, traditional types may be more accurate. If you're worried, have a frank discussion with your doctor before scheduling the scan. If an open MRI is not an option, mild sedation usually is.

Arrange for a health buddy (human or otherwise)

It always helps to have a hand to hold, but if your spouse or friend isn't available, ask the facility if it can supply a paw. A study at Monmouth Medical Center in New Jersey found that interacting with a therapy dog for 15 minutes a half hour before an MRI was so effective at calming patients that the researchers suggested it could replace sedatives.

Health...The Reader's Digest VERSION

Empty your bladder

Since you'll have to remain motionless for up to an hour, never load up on coffee or other liquids before a scan.

Finish a good book

Some facilities have special headsets for viewing or listening to entertainment while being scanned. Check beforehand. If audiobooks are an option, pick up the latest from your favorite author but save the final, riveting chapters for the MRI.

Don't open your eyes

That's when many people start losing it, especially in a closed unit. To make sure you're not tempted, bring along an eye pillow. Even better, scent it with lavender, which is a natural relaxant.

BREATHE LIKE THIS Anxiety builds when you're not breathing enough. This spikes heart rate, deprives the brain of oxygen (essential for rational thought), and makes you feel out of control. To keep this from happening during an MRI, do this:

1. *Exhale thoroughly.*

2. *Inhale through your nose for 3 seconds.*

3. *Purse your lips and exhale to a count of 10 (or however long you can) while letting your cheeks puff. Get every last bit of air out.*

4. *Repeat until you're calm.*

The long exhale ensures that the next inhale is automatically deeper, explains by Al Lee, coauthor of *Perfect Breathing*. This counters the tendency to take short, shallow breaths when you're scared. Practice this exercise beforehand.

Handle an overseas
health emergency

True story. We were on a cruise in the South Pacific when a passenger fell gravely ill. He was taken to a hospital at the next port, but because he needed a blood transfusion and conditions there were deplorable, his wife had him airlifted to New Zealand. Fortunately, he survived, but the $50,000 medical bill nearly killed him. Which goes to prove, Montezuma's revenge is the least of your worries when traveling abroad. Be prepared.

Check your health coverage

Call your healthcare provider to determine what, if any, coverage you have outside the country. If it extends to your destination, be sure to take your insurance ID card and spare claim forms with you. If your coverage is limited (or nonexistent, as is the case with Medicare and Medicaid), absolutely purchase travel medical insurance. Ask your current provider or travel agent for recommendations. Since it's short-term, it's relatively inexpensive.

Evacuate or repatriate?

Medical evacuation is one of the most important components of a travel health policy. It typically covers transportation to the nearest medical facility that can provide appropriate care. It's ideal, however, if medical *repatriation* is also covered. This means that if you'd rather not be treated at Nairobi General, you'll be flown to the hospital of your choice or even home. MedjetAssist is one service that specializes in this, with short-term memberships starting at $95 (medjetassist.com).

Be your own mobile medical file

To speed diagnosis and treatment in a foreign land, keep all your vital health information handy (for example, blood type, allergies, medications, preexisting conditions). Your doctor's office can supply a copy, or there's a 99-cent mobile phone app called "In Case of Emergency" that ensures it's always in your pocket or purse. Another option is a paid service such as MedicAlert (medicalert.org), which stores and sends info when needed.

Learn the 911 equivalent

Most people assume 911 works internationally, but it doesn't. In Hong Kong, for instance, the emergency number is 999, in Australia 000, and throughout the European Union 112. Look up the number for your destination on the U.S. State Department's country guide (travel.state.gov) and program it into your phone.

When in doubt, call the embassy

The State Department maintains embassies, consulates, and diplomatic missions in most major cities and countries. They're your safety net when traveling abroad. Find contact information for every one at usembassy.gov or by downloading the State Department's free Smart Traveler phone app.

DON'T WORRY, BE APPY Download the following and you'll be able to do everything from soothe a toothache to survive a quake:

▸▸ **mPassport:** Find English-speaking doctors and dentists in 180 countries, plus pharmacies and emergency services. Even translates. Thirty-day subscriptions cost $9.95 (mpassport.com).

▸▸ **Pocket First Aid & CPR:** Put together by the American Heart Association, this $3.99 app helped a victim of the Haiti earthquake stay alive for 64 hours under rubble. It also allows you to create your own medical-records profile (jive.me/apps/firstaid).

▸▸ **Google Translate:** Speak or type your question or statement (such as "I need a doctor") and you'll get an automatic visual (and sometimes also audio) translation. Fifty-eight different languages are covered so far (free at your favorite apps store).

Make these health moves in
your
4Os

What	When
Routine checks/exams	
Complete physical	Every 1 to 3 years
Blood pressure	Every 6 months
Cholesterol	Every 2 years
Blood glucose	Every 3 years
Eyesight	Every 2 to 4 years
Teeth	Twice yearly
Hearing	At least once this decade
Body mass index (BMI)	Every 6 months
Skin cancer	Annually
Testicular cancer	Monthly self-exam
Prostate specific antigen (PSA)	Periodically; ask your doctor
Digital rectal	Annually > 45 *(if at risk)*
Colonoscopy	Once per decade *(if at risk, ask your doctor)*
Mammogram	Annually *(okay to wait until age 50)*
Pelvic exam/Pap test	Every 2 to 3 years
Thyroid	Every 5 years

Health... The Reader's Digest VERSION

For many this is the wake-up decade. The number on the bathroom scale is higher than ever, a routine medical exam comes back positive, or a family member or friend is unexpectedly hospitalized. The good news is, we're all remarkably resilient. If your health hasn't been a priority through the first half of life, now is the time to make your comeback.

Inoculations

Influenza	Annually
Tetanus-diphtheria	Once per decade
Others	If missed in prior decades (see page 42)

General

Find a cardiologist.	Heart disease is the number one killer of men in their forties.
Go low-impact.	Hang up the running shoes and switch to joint-friendly workouts.
Adopt a dog.	Pets lower blood pressure.
Prioritize happiness.	Risk of depression is high.
Eat smarter.	Metabolism is still declining.
Get more calcium/vitamin D.	It boosts bone health, especially for women.

Assess the health of
your workplace

Each of us gets sick of working every now and then. But if your symptoms go beyond ordinary stress to actual feelings of illness, it's time to conduct a thorough job review.

Is anyone else feeling this way?
Ask your coworkers. If others are experiencing headaches, burning eyes, respiratory problems, itching, dizziness, nausea, chronic fatigue, or other discomforts that coincide with the workday, it may be a case of Sick Building Syndrome. This can stem from inadequate ventilation or chemical/biological contaminants. Take your evidence to HR or the boss, but couch your complaint in terms of lowered productivity and sick days to get more immediate attention.

Is there secondhand smoke?
If so, then your job is really killing you. Depending on your exposure, passive smoke can increase the risk of lung cancer by 24 to 100 percent. And cigarettes aren't the only source. Wood smoke from fireplaces and stoves raise the odds of lung disease, too.

Can I hear myself think?
A noisy work environment, where you must raise your voice to be heard, makes heart trouble three to four times more likely. It raises diastolic blood pressure, which means arteries never relax between heartbeats and blood flow is chronically constricted. If possible, wear noise-canceling headphones or earplugs.

Am I sitting all day?
Doing so for more than six hours per day raises your chance of dying by 18 percent (for men) and 37 percent (for women)

compared with those who sit less than three hours daily. Frequent breaks help, but what's even better is raising your workstation. Standing burns calories, fights disease, and improves concentration and productivity.

Do others share my workspace?

If your cubicle isn't really *your* cubicle, then start every shift by disinfecting with antibacterial wipes the desk, keyboard, phone, armrests, and anything else you touch.

Do I have access to fresh air and natural light?

If so, turn off the overhead fluorescents (a possible headache trigger) and open the window when possible. If you're trapped, decorate your workspace with peace lily, Gerbera daisies, chrysanthemums, or bamboo palms. In a NASA study these were among the best indoor plants at filtering formaldehyde, benzene, and trichloroethylene from the air. These chemicals can be generated by paint, carpeting, and machinery.

Do I have a company phone?

It may seem like a bonus, but if your boss considers it his 24/7 hotline to you, it can blur boundaries between home and work, leaving you stressed and your health compromised. Turn it off and return calls when *you're* available.

JUST HOW CRAZED ARE YOU AT WORK? Here's an easy way to tell: Instead of a watch, wear a heart-rate monitor. It'll supply an ongoing display of the stress of your workday. You can even set the upper-limit alarm to quietly beep when your pulse rises above a certain point. Over time you'll learn who and what sets you off and, more important, how to step back, take a deep breath, and actually lower your pulse.

Manage an
aging parent

Nearly 10 million American adults over 50 are caring for aging parents. What's ironic is that in their well-intentioned efforts to safeguard Mom and Dad's health, they're often compromising their own. Nearly one-third of these caregivers report stress, anxiety, or depression, and studies also link the process to weight gain and lower overall levels of self-care. If you're doing this job now or anticipating it in the near future, here's how to minimize the wear-and-tear.

Get Nana wired
Communication is the key to managing this life stage, and nothing makes it easier than the Internet. E-mail, video chat (with doctors, no less), photo sharing, Google, and the old standby Solitaire can all help the elderly feel less alone. Be sure to consider tablet devices such as the Apple iPad. Many seniors prefer these over traditional computers and even mobile phones because of their size and ease of use.

Work out the legal stuff
End-of-life issues are complicated, and laws differ by state, so consult a lawyer personally about "advance directives." These include living wills, medical powers of attorney, organ donation, and do-not-resuscitate orders. Granted, these are uncomfortable discussions to have, but a lawyer will facilitate them and ensure there are no legal hassles.

Become a health buddy
Join your mom for medical checkups (or at least talk to her doctor or nurse by phone afterward) to be sure nothing is overlooked. Being fully informed will help ease your worry and better prepare you to take action when necessary. In addition,

monitor her meds for side effects and use reliable sources on the Internet to help stay on top of her conditions (websites ending in .org, .gov, and .edu are most trustworthy). Seniors tend to have blind faith in doctors and healthcare. You need to be their watchdog.

Muster plenty of troops

According to the National Center on Caregiving, "most caregivers are ill-prepared for their role and provide care with little or no support." There are three basic resources to tap:

1. *Family: If you have siblings in the area, divvy up the duties. Ask your spouse or the grandkids to help, too. Having everyone pitch in will ease the burden while making Pappy feel well loved.*

2. *Neighbors: Ask your Facebook friends if they know anyone in the area who'd be willing to pick up groceries or drive Mom to the hairdresser when you can't. There are lots of people looking to do good deeds. You just have to find them.*

3. *Public services: The U.S. Administration on Aging assists seniors nationwide with a variety of free programs. Use its Eldercare Locator at eldercare.gov to find the nearest office. Don't overlook Mom's church, either. Call the pastor to see if it has any charitable services she can take advantage of.*

Keep this in mind

Some of the best advice we ever got about coping with the challenges of eldercare comes from educator Angela Lunde at the Mayo Clinic. "Blame the disease, not the person, when caregiving gets frustrating," she says. By realizing it's not your mom or dad's fault, you'll be better able to treat them (and yourself) with compassion.

PERSONAL N●TES

{ What can I do to help my parents and family be }
more healthy?

Is genetic testing for you?

Genetic testing is possible for about 2,000 diseases, and more tests are being refined daily. No doubt it'll play a large role in future prevention, diagnosis, and treatment. But for now it's much less black and white than it seems. Not only is the science still developing, but there are also moral, ethical, and psychological issues involved. Although it's tempting to peek at your DNA, especially since home test kits are now available, there are important questions to ask before moving forward.

Why are you considering it?
Curiosity alone shouldn't be the driver. Genetic testing is best done under a doctor's supervision when 1) there's a strong first-degree family history of a disease, 2) there's a risk of a child acquiring a serious affliction, or 3) you have symptoms requiring further diagnosis.

What are you looking for?
If it's a predisposition to cystic fibrosis; sickle cell anemia; or breast, ovarian, or colon cancer, genetic testing is more dependable. But for the vast majority of diseases, the genetic link is either less clear or not established. For example, it's estimated that 90 to 95 percent of all cancers *don't* have an inherited component that strongly affects risk.

Can you afford it?
Conventional genetic testing can cost thousands of dollars and is usually not covered by medical insurance.

How vital is your privacy?
The Genetic Information Nondiscrimination Act of 2008 prevents insurers from denying coverage or charging higher

premiums based on the results of genetic tests. It also doesn't allow larger businesses (above 15 workers) to make employment decisions because of them. But in these days of information proliferation and account hacking, could you cope if something leaked out?

Can you handle the verdict?

Learning you're carrying a potentially deadly gene that you may have passed along to your children is some heavy psychological baggage. A positive result doesn't guarantee development of disease, but it does assure some degree of worry, probably for the rest of your life.

Will you act on the results?

If you'll use a positive result as an impetus to make meaningful lifestyle changes, then knowledge is power. But if you'll likely do nothing or, worse, forgo prevention because you think a negative result is ironclad protection (which it's not), then knowing you're at risk may actually increase your risk.

Are you enough of an expert to make this decision?

Most people aren't. In fact, many doctors don't fully appreciate all the implications of genetic testing. The smartest move if you're serious about moving forward is to meet with a genetic counselor. These specialists will help you answer all the questions we just raised. Find one at the "Find a Genetic Counselor" tool at nsgc.org.

Finding
solutions

When it comes to repairing some health issues and insulating yourself against others, there's a lot you can nail on your own. In that respect, this section is your Home Depot—the land of the personal health handyman. From soothing your various aches and pains to decreasing your risk of diabetes and cancer, each chapter is a separate, well-stocked aisle.

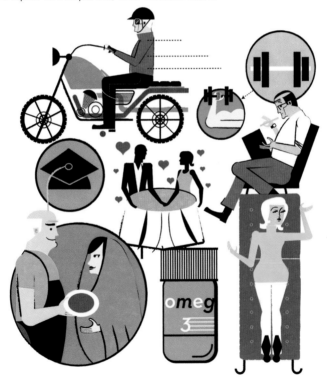

Turn off a
headache

Doctors can replace entire hearts and hips, but when it comes to something as everyday as a headache, they're still often perplexed. That's because there are more than 150 different types, each with unique symptoms, severities, and causes that range from anxiety to allergies, hypertension to hormones, ice cream to orgasms. When it seems like Charlie Watts is drumming in your head, here's how to make him quit.

Have a cup of coffee and two ibuprofen gel caps
Studies point to this combo as providing the fastest and longest-lasting relief from most headaches. The caffeine apparently speeds delivery of the medication, while also shrinking swollen blood vessels in the head. For more debilitating migraines the combination of acetaminophen, aspirin, and caffeine in Excedrin Migraine, for instance, appears to work best.

Become a headhunter
To find the source of your hurt, start keeping a headache journal. This is a simple matter of recording what you were doing in the hours before the pain struck. Meals, mood, time of day, location—note it all, along with how the headache feels and where it's located (temples, sinus, behind the eye, forehead, neck, and so on). Eventually, certain patterns may emerge that point to specific triggers, which can then be avoided.

Stay away from Tyra
Roughly 20 percent of migraine headaches are diet-induced, and it's not just MSG and alcohol that are responsible. A naturally occurring amino acid called tyramine is often to blame. It's especially concentrated in foods that are aged, dried, fermented,

or stored for long periods. Cheese, processed meat, nuts, red wine, and even pickles can be instigators.

Switch off the light

Certain types of flickering or glaring light from fluorescent bulbs, computer monitors, TV screens, and even the sun (in snow or beach conditions) can cause headaches. To minimize the effects, turn off overhead office lighting (or counter it with incandescent table lamps), install antiglare screens, and wear polarized sunglasses outdoors.

See a specialist

The previous steps often help, but if not, don't suffer in silence. A headache, unless its source is the other family members living in your home, does not have to be chronic. Beyond over-the-counters and home remedies, there is expert help available in the form of headache specialists and neurologists. (Ask your doctor for a referral.) There are even some interesting treatments, including Botox facial injections, which promise to make you feel *and* look better!

THE BIG THREE There are three general categories of headaches: tension, migraine, and cluster. *Tension headaches* are the most common. They're caused by anxiety, fatigue, or a stressful environment and make your head feel like it's in one of Suzanne Somers's ThighMasters. *Migraine headaches* are more intense, characterized by throbbing pain, nausea, and hypersensitivity to light and noise. They have assorted triggers, including food, hormones, and weather. *Cluster headaches* are often the most continuously painful, centering on one side of the head or behind an eye. As their name implies, these don't last long (30 to 45 minutes) but recur throughout the day.

Stop the snoring

If your partner sounds like a '69 Mustang with an open throttle when he's "sleeping," then your relationship (and your health) are in serious trouble. Having your rest routinely disturbed by a chronic snorer can lead to arguments, lower libido, resentment, separate bedrooms, and even divorce. Poor sleep is also linked to high blood pressure, stroke, and diabetes. Since it's often difficult to get someone to admit to a snoring problem, let alone see a specialist, here are some sneaky ways you can try to fix it.

Move up last call
Snoring is caused by the vibration of loose throat tissue as air passes over it. Alcohol consumption further relaxes throat muscles and thereby compounds the tendency to snore. Make last call at least two hours before lights out.

Raise the head of the bed
To keep his tongue from flopping back over his airway (hey, you married him), put a 4-inch (10-cm) brick or sturdy block under each leg at the head of the bed. As a beauty bonus for you, it'll reduce facial blood pooling and eye puffiness. It also helps heartburn.

Promote healthy eating
A poor diet not only promotes obesity, which fattens throat tissue and narrows air passages, it can also cause acid reflux, which further inflames that area.

Decongest the area
Allergies and colds are another common cause of snoring. Offer a decongestant before bed or a Breathe Right nasal strip, which helps keep nostrils open while sleeping.

Hide the sleeping pills

If your mate relies on medication to sleep, he may unwittingly be compounding the problem. Such drugs generally work by depressing the central nervous system and further relaxing throat muscles.

Get off his back

Because snoring is compounded by sleeping faceup, try duct-taping or sewing a golf ball to the back of his nightshirt. This will keep him on his side.

Spark an interest in music

According to a *British Medical Journal* study, regularly playing a didgeridoo (a traditional Australian wind instrument) reduces snoring by toning throat muscles. If it turns out the sound of him playing a didgeridoo is even worse than the snoring itself, encourage singing instead. Twenty minutes per day of certain vocal exercises, such as la-la-la and ma-ma-ma, may have the same effect, reports the Mayo Clinic.

Get help if you hear this...

Although these home remedies are often effective, if your partner frequently awakens with a start from his snores or it seems as if his breathing is interrupted, take him to a doctor immediately. He may have sleep apnea, a condition that can damage lungs nearly as much as smoking.

RECORD THE RUMBLING If all else fails, put a mobile phone or tape recorder on your nightstand and press the record button the next time you're awakened by the din. Then play it through your stereo system on continuous loop at high volume when your bed partner is trying to have a little quiet time. He'll get the idea. Plus, his doctor can use the recording to diagnose sleep apnea on his next visit.

Tell if it's impotence
or anxiety

What we're really discussing here is the difference between physical and psychological erectile dysfunction (ED). The former results from a specific problem in the body that prevents the penis from getting hard enough for intercourse, while the latter, which is to blame in up to 20 percent of cases, stems from more elusive mental issues of which boredom can be just one. Since many men find it humiliating to consult a doctor about this, here are a few easy ways to assess if it's a physical problem that requires medical help or a psychological one that could work itself out.

Assess his stress
Anxiety over career, finances, relationships, looks, even kids can distract a man from the task at hand. So if he's been going through a rough patch lately (and drinking more alcohol to cope), then the combination could be what's leaving him limp.

Try something fresh
If you've been making love in the same place at the same time in the same way since the Reagan administration, reserve an out-of-town room at a romantic B&B and by all means pack the Lady Gaga outfit. If the other guests tell you to keep it down, smile and explain that's exactly the problem you're here to cure.

Peek under the sheets
If he's getting solid erections while asleep, then that's firm evidence any performance problems are psychological. If you don't feel like keeping a midnight watch, wrap postage stamps around the base of his penis (no, we're not kidding) and secure

the ends. If they're ripped along the perforation the next morning, everything is still working. If he's not in bed when you wake up, check the post office.

Inspect his seat

If he took up bicycling recently, his saddle might be to blame. Any type of hard or narrow seat that's used for long periods can cause temporary ED by compressing nerves and restricting blood flow. Suggest Lance take a few days off and see if function returns.

Check the medicine cabinet

Certain antidepressants (Prozac, Zoloft), antihistamines (Benadryl, Dramamine), and nonsteroidal anti-inflammatories (Naproxen) can cause erection problems. If he's started taking any of these lately, consult a doctor about alternatives.

See if his heart is still beating

Good erections require good blood flow. That's why impotency can be an early warning sign of heart disease or maybe even diabetes. If your guy has a family history of either or has other risk factors (overweight, smoker), treat the lack of a flagpole as a red flag and get medical attention pronto.

ONE PILL MAKES YOU LARGER All those TV commercials for Viagra, Levitra, and Cialis aren't just marketing hype. A study of nearly 8,000 men found all three improved erectile function and sexual satisfaction after six months of treatment. And in case you were wondering, no other vitamin or herbal supplement has that kind of definitive research behind it.

Make these health moves in
your
50s

What	When
Routine checks/exams	
Complete physical	Every 1 to 3 years
Blood pressure	Every 6 months
Cholesterol	Every 2 years
Blood glucose	Every 3 years
Eyesight	Every 2 to 4 years
Teeth	Twice yearly
Hearing	Every 3 years
Body mass index (BMI)	Every 6 months
Skin cancer	Annually
Prostate specific antigen (PSA)	Periodically; ask your doctor
Digital rectal	Annually
Fecal occult blood	Annually
Sigmoidoscopy	Every 5 years
Colonoscopy	Once per decade
Bone density	Periodically *(if at risk; ask your doctor)*
Mammogram	Annually
Pelvic exam/Pap test	Every 2 to 3 years
Thyroid	Every 5 years

raditionally, this is the best decade of life for many men and women. Career and family pressures have eased, and you have more time, money, and wisdom to appreciate life. Congratulations, you've arrived. Now make sure an unexpected health problem doesn't trigger a premature departure.

Inoculations

Influenza	Annually
Measles/mumps/rubella	Once if born in 1957 or later *(ask doctor)*
Tetanus-diphtheria	Once per decade
Others	If missed in prior decades *(see page 42)*

General

Take up yoga.	Restores flexibility/posture/calm.
Manage midlife changes.	If necessary, consult a specialist.
Eat even smarter.	Metabolism is still declining.
Pursue a passion.	It keeps you young.

Prevent diabetes

Unlike heart attack, stroke, or cancer, diabetes doesn't sound like a killer. But it's the seventh-leading cause of death in the United States, and that's with a bullet. Once you develop it, you've just doubled your risk of dying. Fortunately, while you can be genetically predisposed to diabetes, it's mostly caused by lifestyle factors. In fact, according to diabetes researcher Richard Béliveau, PhD, adopting a healthful lifestyle can prevent up to 90 percent of type-2 cases (and help you manage it better if you already have the disease). Here's your best defense.

Lose 5 to 7 percent of your weight
That's all the fat you need to shave in order to enjoy a nearly 60 percent reduction in risk if you also exercise 150 minutes each week, according to a landmark study sponsored by the National Institutes of Health. It's the most significant step you can take to fight diabetes—one with an even greater effect than the popular antidiabetic drug metformin.

Walk 2½ hours per week
Increased physical activity was one of the ways participants in that previous study reduced their risk of diabetes. It equates to 30 minutes of walking (or other exercise of moderate intensity) five days per week. To stay committed, block off that half hour on your daily schedule as you would any other important appointment.

Go low-cal and low-fat
This was the other way those study participants succeeded. Although it's advice you've probably heard (and tried) many times, here are some new ways to make it stick.

Eat a big brinner.

People who eat breakfast are 35 to 50 percent less likely to become overweight and develop insulin resistance. For energy balance it also helps to make your first meal of the day your biggest meal of the day (call it "brinner"). Too rushed in the morning? Fill your mug with a healthful coffee smoothie. Blend together 1 cup cold, strong-brewed coffee; 1 banana; 1 cup low-fat vanilla yogurt; 1 cup ice; and if desired, one packet of zero-calorie sweetener.

›› **Make friends with fiber.** *A diet rich in whole grains, fruits, and vegetables can lower your diabetic risk by up to 34 percent.*

›› **Swear off soda.** *Just one a day, whether regular or diet, has been linked to a 44 percent greater chance of developing metabolic syndrome, a collection of risk factors for diabetes and cardiovascular disease.*

›› **Watch out for the worst fats.** *That would be saturated and trans fat. Both are prevalent in fast food. Eating just two burgers with fries every week can jack up your odds of metabolic syndrome by as much as 50 percent.*

Be happy

Depression not only makes it less likely you'll exercise and eat well, it also appears to be a stand-alone risk factor for diabetes. In a Stanford University study it altered body chemistry in ways that raised insulin resistance 23 percent among women.

THE DIABETES 11 Based on the latest research gathered by the American Diabetes Association, here are the 11 best foods for fighting this disease. They're all rich in calcium, potassium, fiber, magnesium, and vitamins A, C and E—the nutrients that appear to pack the most punch. (Note that the ADA recommends getting them through food, not supplements.)

▸▸ Beans

▸▸ Dark leafy greens

▸▸ Citrus fruit

▸▸ Sweet potatoes

▸▸ Berries

▸▸ Tomatoes

▸▸ Fish (high in omega-3 fatty acids, such as salmon)

▸▸ Whole grains

▸▸ Nuts

▸▸ Skim milk

▸▸ Fat-free yogurt

PERSONAL NOTES

{ What will I do today to **prevent** diabetes
or heart disease in the future? }

Beat the blues
(without medicine)

These days everybody wants to be happy all the time. But humans just weren't designed to live that way. It's like vacation. In order to fully appreciate the sweetness of the beach, you need a job that continually puts sand in your suit. So the key strategy for weathering bad moods is simply realizing they're a natural part of life that will ultimately make you feel happier by comparison. That being said, if you tend to feel down more than up, you might have depression, a real disease. Here are some natural solutions for bad moods and their more serious counterpart.

Sweat up a smile
Exercise releases feel-good hormones called endorphins that appear to be even more potent than antidepressants. Duke University researchers found that people with major depressive disorders not only benefited more from exercise than those taking Zoloft but also had significantly fewer relapses. Any type of exercise will do. Just move.

Make a habit out of breaking habits
Psychologist Douglas Newburg, PhD, estimates that 99 percent of most adults' lives are habit and routine. In fact, since the brain is an expensive organ to operate metabolically (meaning, it uses lots of fuel), its tendency is to run on autopilot. But being in a rut like that can get depressing. To break out, try to do one thing differently every day. Shop at a new grocery store. Listen

to another radio station in the car. Over time you'll get addicted to the way these little deviations wake you up and freshen your outlook.

Shift from a fixed to a growth mindset
Many depressed people feel they're imprisoned by their personalities, that they are who they are and there's nothing they can do about it. Wrong. "Yes, we have failures and hit obstacles, but we're all works in progress," says Carol Dweck, PhD, a Stanford University professor of psychology. She suggests viewing your next setback as a learning opportunity rather than as fate.

Fight D with D
Chronic vitamin D deficiency can make you sadder than necessary. To check on yours, ask your doctor to add a vitamin D analysis to your next blood test. If your level is low, eat more D-rich foods or spend additional time in the sunshine (or in a room lit by full-spectrum bulbs).

Pet a pet
Sadness often arises from feeling alone and unloved. But pets, since they make you the center of their universe, instantly solve that. When, for instance, was the last time anyone peed with joy when you came home from work? 'Nuff said.

> **SWISS MISS FOR BLISS** Sometimes all it takes to turn the corner on a dour mood is a single moment of quiet joy. According to Alan Hirsch, MD at the Smell & Taste Treatment Center and Research Foundation, hot chocolate does this best. Not only does the taste of chocolate boost mood because of its deep-seated reward and comfort connotations, but in liquid form its smell also tickles olfactory bulbs and compounds these effects.

Check for
skin cancer

Quick quiz: What's the most common type of cancer in the United States? Answer: It isn't breast or lung cancer, which attract most of the charity events and press. Rather, it's skin cancer, which affects more than two million Americans annually—over 60,000 of whom are diagnosed with the deadliest variety (melanoma). Unlike most other diseases, however, you don't need any invasive or expensive tests to catch this one early. At least at the outset, you can be your own dermatologist.

Strip for someone
You can't do a thorough job of this yourself, so recruit your spouse or someone you'd like to know better. Take off all your clothes and, in a well-lit room, have them examine every inch of you. Look for odd-shaped moles or oversized freckles. Include your scalp, between your fingers and toes, and even in those places where the sun rarely goes. (Then, by all means, return the favor.)

Do the ABCD test
Moles should be examined according to the following criteria: asymmetry (does one half match the other?), border irregularity (are the edges jagged?), color (is it uniform?), and diameter (is it more than a quarter inch wide?) If anything looks suspicious, see a doctor.

Look beyond the alphabet
Other warning signs in or around a mole include redness, swelling, itchiness, tenderness, pain, oozing, and bleeding. All are signals to consult an expert as well.

Take some photos

If you're at high risk for skin cancer (or just really bored), you can photograph certain moles to better monitor their evolution. These can even be e-mailed to your dermatologist for a quick opinion.

Inspect your car, inspect yourself

Use the inspection sticker on your car's windshield as an annual reminder to get yourself inspected by a dermatologist. Each year when your vehicle comes due, so do you. In the interim conduct your own amateur inspection every two to three months as outlined above.

Carry a dermatologist in your pocket

Skin Scan is a $9.99 iPhone/iPad app that scans, analyzes, and then archives your moles. Simply take a clear photograph of the skin lesion and let the app use "mathematical algorithms and fractal analysis" to gauge whether it's low, medium, or high risk. It even comes with a handy list of nearby doctors to consult.

GOOD BOY If your dog is continually sniffing or licking a part of your body, don't shoo him away. He may be trying to tell you something. Some dogs can actually smell cancer and are being used in research labs to do so. If the spot he's concerned with looks suspicious, get it checked (and give him a treat).

Get rid of a cold

The common cold is responsible for more doctor visits in the United States than any other illness. The reason colds are so difficult to cure is because more than 200 distinct viruses are to blame. And 20 to 30 percent of colds have no known cause. To help unclog our healthcare system, here are some tips on unclogging yourself.

Make sure it's a cold
If you have swollen glands, severe sinus pain, a mucus-producing cough, and/or high fever, you could have something worse and you *should* consult a doctor. Conversely, if you have a runny nose, itchy eyes, and other minor coldlike symptoms that recur frequently or seasonally, you may have allergies. Know thy enemy.

For temporary relief, take this
The over-the-counter adult decongestant most recommended by pharmacists is Sudafed, according to a survey by the American Pharmacists Association. While no OTC med will cure a cold, this one is particularly effective at drying up mucus and preventing it from dripping into your throat and lungs, where it can compound the problem. If you prefer a nasal decongestant, Ocean Saline is the pharmacists' top choice.

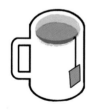

Get into a green routine
Freshly brewed green tea contains a high concentration of EGCG, a natural chemical compound that researchers have found inhibits the replication of the adenovirus cold bug. If swigged at the onset of symptoms, the cold's duration may be shortened.

Have chicken soup (for breakfast)
As the wives' tale goes, feed that cold. One small study found that a 1,200-calorie breakfast boosts blood levels of antiviral

agents by 450 percent, which is nothing to sniff at. But instead of eating the usual morning fare, try substituting chicken soup (Starclucks?). Some research suggests that it may reduce the inflammation that causes cold symptoms.

Rest rather than exercise
Although regular exercise strengthens immunity, it's not clear whether it helps chase a cold. A Ball State University study found little difference in cold duration between those who worked out while sick and those who didn't. Because there's a risk of intensifying illness if you exercise too hard with a cold, it's probably smarter to take a few days off. In fact, sleep is the body's preferred way to repair itself.

Play a video game
This is a long shot, but there is some evidence that a short bout of manageable stress, like people typically experience when playing video games, floods the body with disease-fighting proteins. So take one Xbox and call us in the morning.

SUPPLEMENTS FOR SNIFFLES: DO THEY WORK? There are more of them for sale than there are tissues in a box. But are they effective? Here's the verdict from the National Institute of Allergy and Infectious Diseases on the most popular alternative remedies:

▸▸ **Echinacea:** Three big studies found no effect.

▸▸ **Vitamin C:** No clear evidence of any benefit.

▸▸ **Zinc:** May slightly reduce symptoms/duration.

PERSONAL N●TES

{ What are my favorite **home remedies?** }

Quit smoking

Finished. Free. Finally. Getting through the first week is the key. Research shows that within two days of swearing off, half of all quitters are lighting up. And by the end of that initial week, two-thirds are back to reaching for a pack. These strategies focus on this crucial period when mental and physical withdrawal symptoms peak and you're most weak.

Put thoughts of cold turkey on ice

The sad fact is that only 4 to 7 percent of smokers are able to quit without any help, either emotional or medical. That's because smoking isn't just a bad habit; it's an addiction. Admit you need assistance.

Line up someone to lean on

Just as with exercise and weight loss, staying with a commitment is easier if there's someone to support and encourage you. Set a quit date, then schedule an appointment with your doctor, a cognitive behavioral therapist, or a smoking-cessation support group during those first few days. Or visit naquitline.org to find a telephone hotline in your state that's manned by experts adept at talking people down off their Camels. One study found that 33 percent of those who used these lines were still smoke-free after 12 months compared to just 5 percent of those who didn't use any help at all.

Line up some nicotine to wean on

Nicotine-replacement therapy (NRT) supplies the drug you crave in alternative ways, thereby blunting physical withdrawal symptoms. FDA-approved NRTs include gum, lozenges, inhalers, nasal sprays, and patches, all with varying degrees of effectiveness. If you're confused by the options, ask your doctor about these as well as prescription medications.

Exercise for five minutes
Whenever the urge hits to go outside for a smoke, take a leisurely 300-second walk. No matter how out of shape you are, you can manage this. Or if there's an exercise bike turned clothes hanger in the house, hop on that for five minutes. The activity will distract you from your craving, reduce stress (a smoking trigger), and counter weight gain (a common side effect of quitting).

Pat yourself on the back frequently
Within 20 minutes of stubbing out that last butt, your heart rate and blood pressure drop. After 12 hours the carbon monoxide in your bloodstream clears. And by the end of the first day, your risk of heart attack is lower. Your circulation is also improving, your sense of taste and smell is returning, and your breathing is better (not to mention your breath). Congratulate yourself (repeatedly) on the significant progress you're making. Quitting is the single best thing you can do for your health.

SMOKED MEAT: ANOTHER SMOKING GUN Researchers at the Harvard School of Public Health found that processed meat (smoked, cured, salted, and otherwise preserved) contains carcinogens, or potentially cancer-causing compounds. Eating processed meats also raises the risk of heart disease by 42 percent and type 2 diabetes by 19 percent. There is good news, though. This research, which spanned 20 studies and 1.2 million participants, did not find an increased risk from eating *unprocessed* red meat, such as beef, pork, and lamb.

PERSONAL N●TES

{ What unhealthy **habits** am I going to try and give up—
and how am I going to do it? }

Extinguish heartburn

Ever hear of hydrochloric acid? It's used to remove rust from steel and dissolve rock during well drilling. It's also the chief ingredient in stomach acid, which explains how it's possible to digest your mother-in-law's holiday rump roast. Sometimes, however, this corrosive acid splashes up into your esophagus, where it's felt as a burning sensation and can do a lot of damage. If allowed to become chronic, it can even cause cancer. Let's get this under control now.

Gauge the frequency of your burn
For most people heartburn or acid indigestion is an uncomfortable nuisance resulting from an occasional indulgence. But for others it's an ongoing curse stemming from a malfunction in the valvelike muscle linking the stomach with the esophagus. If your heartburn is frequent (more than twice weekly) and severe, you may have that second condition, which is called gastroesophageal reflux disease (GERD).

Flush out the fat
Most people treat their stomachs with less regard than their toilets, throwing in all kinds of junk, then wondering why things keep backing up. We don't mean to be insensitive to your plumbing woes, but eating smarter (fewer fatty foods/ more fiber), having smaller meals, not lying down for three hours following a meal, and losing weight is the simplest way to reduce episodes of heartburn and GERD. Experiment to find your trigger foods (they're not the same for everybody), and remember that excess pounds put excess pressure on that stomach-esophagus intersection.

Let Mother Nature be your nurse
There are lots of home remedies for heartburn. Although not long-term solutions, many can provide temporary relief and are

worth a try. Chewing gum, for example, produces more saliva, which dilutes acidic backwash. Ginger, either the candied variety or in tea, has been used as a stomach soother for centuries. And although the exact reasons are unclear, a teaspoon of yellow mustard or a couple almonds after a meal works for some sufferers. The remedy doesn't have to be herbal, either. Some studies have found that elevating the head of your bed 6 to 9 inches (15 to 23 cm) and sleeping on your left side significantly reduces nighttime reflux, as does avoiding sleeping pills.

Call in the pharmacy

Although drugs called PPIs (proton-pump inhibitors) are very effective, they can shut down stomach-acid production too much if taken for long periods. Even over-the-counter versions, like Prilosec and Prevacid, should be used cautiously. Better to start treatment with milder OTC medications, such as antacids (Tums, Rolaids, Mylanta), and then if there's no relief, step up to acid blockers, like Pepcid AC, Zantac, or Tagamet. If you're still suffering, ask your doctor about those PPIs or a new diagnostic technique called CLE, in which a tiny microscope is lowered into the esophagus to better assess the situation.

---

3 MYTHS DEBUNKED

▸▸ **Heartburn medication should always be taken after a meal:**
You may be able to head off heartburn entirely if you take an acid blocker a half hour *before* eating food that normally causes indigestion.

▸▸ **Drinking milk dampens the fire:** It doesn't have any effect on heartburn, and if you're swigging some with a higher fat content, it may actually provoke it.

▸▸ **Heartburn damages the heart:** Although symptoms are sometimes felt in the chest area, acid backup does not extend to your ticker.

Soothe cranky joints

Do you wake up every morning feeling like the Tin Man in the *Wizard of Oz?* If so, don't believe for a minute that this, like wrinkles and wraparounds, is an inevitable part of growing old. Instead of resigning yourself to Aleve for the rest of your life, here's a well-oiled, medication-free plan for feeling young again.

Make friends with your fascia

Under your skin you wear a suit of interconnected tendons and tissue called fascia. With maturity and mistreatment this suit can begin to feel a few sizes too small, as evidenced by the constricted appearance of so many little old ladies and men. This is all reversible, however, with some appropriate tailoring. First, keep your fascia well hydrated by drinking plenty of water. Otherwise, it actually starts to look like beef jerky. Next, start doing yoga to gradually stretch the fibers in this suit. Sign up for a free introductory class at a local studio, or learn the simple 10-minute Sun Salutation series outlined on page 24.

Roll it away

Try this simple experiment for one week. Each day while you're sitting at your desk or on the sofa, slowly roll your head and neck three times clockwise and three times counterclockwise. At first you'll hear lots of crackling, which is normal, but by the end of the week, these noises will mostly disappear. Regular yoga practices quiet and loosen your entire body this same way. Find similar soothing moves for the joints that are bothering you most, and do them each day.

Live low-impact

Just like a car's suspension, your fascial system gets creaky over time. The vibrations from all the roads we travel and the potholes we hit take their toll. So minimize the damage by avoiding repetitive high-impact activities like running or jumping on hard surfaces. Stay aerobically fit with low-impact sports, such as walking, swimming, and bicycling.

Tuna out the pain

While research on glucosamine, chondroitin, SAM-e, vitamin E, and other natural joint-pain relievers remains inconclusive, there is one supplement that appears to be effective. Studies show that omega-3 fatty acids (fish oil) reduce inflammation in joints and throughout the body, which benefits the heart. Salmon, mackerel, and tuna are great natural sources.

Reevaluate cholesterol medication

Joint pain is a common side effect of some cholesterol-lowering drugs. So if your aches arrived with your new prescription, call your doctor.

MATTRESS MATTERS If your current mattress was bought in the 20th century, it could be the reason why you're feeling so battle weary. Cornell sleep expert James B. Maas, PhD, recommends buying a new one at least every decade. Forgotten how old yours is? "If you've recently had a better night's sleep in a hotel or even a tent, it is probably shot," he says. "Find a new one that keeps your head, neck, and spine aligned as if you were standing." Oh, and write an expiration date of 10 years in the future on the tag so you'll know when to replace it.

End **knee pain** pronto

If your knees ache so much that even getting down on them to pray for help is out of the question, here are some potentially heaven-sent solutions.

Get a 4-for-1 deal
For every pound of weight you lose, the stress on your knees drops fourfold. For example, losing 5 pounds lightens their load by the equivalent of 20 pounds, 10 by 40, 15 by 60, and so on. Weight loss is the simplest, most effective thing you can do to pull your joints back from their aching point.

Examine your sole
Look at the bottoms of your favorite shoes. If they're worn consistently along the outsides (or insides), then the natural roll of your feet while you walk or run may be twisting your knees. A podiatrist, or foot doctor, can design shoe inserts called orthotics to balance things out. Shoes themselves can also cause knee trouble. On days when you ache, note which ones you were wearing. Sometimes alleviating the pain is as simple as (yes!) going shopping for new ones.

Do some quad pumps
If you spend most of the day seated and it's a dull knee ache that's plaguing you, your joints may not be getting enough lubrication (such as blood, oxygen, and nutrients). While seated, extend your legs with heels on the floor, contract both thigh muscles for a few seconds, then release and repeat 11 more times. Get into the habit of also doing this exercise during meetings, subway rides, flights, and long dinners.

Make this a mealtime standard
Studies show that three of the best foods for your knees are soy, fish, and fruit. The first two supply anti-inflammatory

compounds, while the last provides vitamin C, all of which nourish the knee. Try combining the trio in a meal. Have salmon topped with kiwi/orange/mango salsa and a glass of soy milk. Or head to your nearest Japanese restaurant and order mackerel, tuna, and salmon sashimi with edamame (soy beans) on the side.

Exercise more softly

You don't have to beat your body up to get a good workout. Brisk walking, swimming, and bicycling are low-impact activities that are kind to knees. If you're cycling, just remember to have your bike professionally fitted at a bike shop and, whenever you're exercising outdoors, cover your knees when temperatures dip below 60°F (16°C).

Recipe for Relief

For those days when you overdo it (and get a headache to boot), follow this easy recipe for scoring some relief:

1. *Ingredients/Supplies*

    ▸▸ 1 1/2 cups water

    ▸▸ 1/2 cup rubbing alcohol

    ▸▸ 1 zipper-seal plastic freezer bag (quart size)

2. *Pour water and alcohol into bag, seal, and freeze. The alcohol will keep the water from completely freezing, leaving you with a moldable slush that conforms perfectly to knees (and foreheads).*

3. *Lean back, say Ahhh.*

Prevent Alzheimer's

There's a retired guy in our neighborhood who we've known for years. On summer evenings he'd sit on his porch listening to the Phillies. But the last time we stopped to chat, he didn't know the score or even who we were. His wife told us he'd been diagnosed with Alzheimer's. This debilitating disease is now the sixth leading cause of death in the United States and the only one in the top 10 that cannot be slowed or cured. But that doesn't mean we're defenseless. Here's the best stay-sharp plan we know.

Don't waste money on brain boosters

Lots of vitamins and supplements claim to enhance brain health, but don't swallow that hype. Products that contain a variety of brain-boosting herbs and even those that deliver just one, like ginkgo biloba, have little if any supporting research, says brain expert Thomas Crook III, PhD.

Strengthen the heart; protect the brain

The brain is a highly vascular organ, meaning it's full of blood vessels. When you're concentrating, it can use up to 50 percent of the body's total available fuel and oxygen. That means anything that's beneficial for the heart and circulatory system is also good for the brain. Exercising, eating less saturated fat and more fruits and vegetables, not smoking, controlling cholesterol...the prescription isn't any different. In fact, Alzheimer's may be a side effect of heart disease.

Befriend your local fishmonger

Eating three servings of fish per week may lower your risk of Alzheimer's by 50 percent. Scientists believe this is due to specific compounds called omega-3 fatty acids. These bolster the cardiovascular system and promote brain growth and development. (One of these compounds, DHA, is actually abundant in mother's milk.) The latest thinking, however, is that omega-3s are best utilized by the body when ingested naturally rather than as supplements.

Be a lifelong learner
Whether you're studying a second language, researching a topic on the Internet, or just doing the Sunday crossword, the effort involved is mental exercise. Learning is Zumba for the brain.

Think about what you drink
To keep your brain functioning at a high level, drink plenty of water. However, there's no proven benefit to special concoctions such as SmartWater. There is some evidence that caffeine, in moderation, may be protective of memory. And when it comes to alcohol, one large study found that those who downed more than 14 drinks per week suffered a 1.6 percent reduction in relative brain volume.

Sleep eight to nine hours nightly
Your brain is still on while your body is off. It's operating at a maintenance and restorative level that's essential to long-term function and health. Being well rested is not just a way to be productive the next day but also well into the future.

A BRAIN ON TOP OF ITS GAME

20 to 25 percent ▸▸ The amount of total blood volume delivered to the brain with every heartbeat

100 billion ▸▸ The number of nerve cells or neurons in an adult brain

100 trillion ▸▸ The number of connection points or synapses between those cells (the so-called neuron forest)

Put a stop to
cold sores

Although they're medically insignificant, these little devils can cause a great deal of personal hell because they're so visible and unsightly. And because cold sores often are sparked by stress, they always seem to appear at the worst possible times (important presentations, meetings, vacations, dates). Unfortunately, there's no cure for the herpes simplex viruses that causes these bothersome blisters, but their frequency and duration can be managed quite well. Assuming you're already carrying the virus (as 50 to 80 percent of adult Americans are), here's how to be a more successful sore loser.

Avoid pulling the typical triggers

The virus that causes cold sores lies dormant until something awakens it. These triggers include prolonged sun exposure (without using a lip balm of SPF 15 or higher), lack of sleep, anxiety, colds and flu, and any sort of lip trauma (so go easy on the kissing, lover). There is also some evidence that arginine, an amino acid found in shellfish, spinach, sesame seeds, turkey, and many other foods causes them. To see if you're sensitive, review your diet in the days before an outbreak.

Put it on ice

As soon as you feel a lip tingle or itch, wrap an ice cube in a thin towel and hold it on the spot for a few minutes. Do this repeatedly for one and a half to two hours and the sore may either never blossom or be less severe.

Find your best defense

There are lots of home remedies with some supporting research that may or may not work for you. When an outbreak seems imminent or is in progress, try taking aspirin (125 mg daily), lysine (1,000 to 3,000 mg daily), echinacea (1,200 mg daily), quercetin (1,000 mg daily), or applying lemon balm ointment. Don't do everything at once, though. Use a process of elimination.

Arm yourself with antivirals

If you don't want to waste time experimenting with home remedies, ask your doctor or dermatologist about oral and topical prescription medications that can minimize outbreaks and their severity. These include valacyclovir (Valtrex), famciclovir (Famvir), acyclovir (Zovirax), and penciclovir (Denavir). An over-the-counter cream with some positive supporting research is docosanol (Abreva).

Wait it out

The frequency of outbreaks tends to decrease with age, so if you can use the previous strategies to keep them at bay, by age 35 or so they should become less of a worry.

KEEP YOUR SISTER-IN-LAW AWAY

Q: Most people acquire oral herpes as children. How do they get it?

A: A kiss from a friend or relative, whether they're symptomatic at the time or not.

Never suffer
from osteoporosis

By the time you're 18 (for women) or 20 (for men), you have 85 to 90 percent of the bone mass you'll have for life. Your job then becomes one of maintenance. If you're not careful, you can lose 0.6 to 1.0 percent of your bone density every year, which in time can leave your skeleton so brittle that sneezing could cause a fracture. Although osteoporosis has traditionally been regarded as a postmenopausal women's disease, 20 percent of sufferers are men. But relax. If you're smart, there's no need to ever get bent out of shape.

Bone up on family history
Osteoporosis has a large genetic component. If your parents and/or grandparents are alive, encourage them to have a bone mineral density (BMD) test at their next medical checkup. If they've passed away, look for telltale signs of osteoporosis (height loss, forward-curving spine) in photos.

Calculate your calcium
Bone is living tissue, and calcium is the mineral that sustains it. Adults need 1,000 mg (under age 50) to 1,200 mg (over age 50) daily. Ideally, this should come from a mix of natural sources such as dairy, broccoli, beans, tofu, and dark, leafy greens. (A recent study in the *British Medical Journal* suggests calcium supplements raise the risk of heart attacks.) Periodic blood and urine tests can be done to monitor levels.

Mobilize your D-fense
Calcium may be the major construction material in bone, but vitamin D is the foreman that makes sure it's being efficiently used. Adults need 400 to 800 IU (under age 50) and 800 to 1,000 IU (over age 50) daily. The easiest way to get your dose is by

spending 10 to 15 minutes outdoors each day before applying sunscreen. To see how strong your D-fense is, ask your doctor to have it measured on your next blood test.

Exercise smarter

There are two types of exercise that benefit bone most. The first is weight-bearing activity, like walking and tennis, which utilizes the skeleton for support and impact-resistance. (Non-weight-bearing activities, like swimming and bicycling, do not.) The second type is resistance training, which for most people means lifting weights. In fact, bone responds just like muscle does to weight lifting, becoming bigger, denser, and stronger.

Be wary of these

According to the National Osteoporosis Foundation, ingesting too much protein, sodium, and soda may promote calcium and bone loss. Studies point to high-protein fad diets and cola drinks in particular.

BUILD BETTER BALANCE WITH ONE MOVE There's an important component of fitness beyond strength, endurance, and flexibility that most people neglect. It's balance, and it becomes increasingly vital with age. The evidence? A shocking 24 percent of hip-fracture patients over 50 die in the year following their fracture. Whether you have osteoporosis or not, preventing a fall is a smart health move. Hone it by making this simple exercise a regular part of your workout:

Stand with a wall or other sturdy object on your left, pick a stationary focal point directly ahead, and slowly raise your right leg until the knee is bent at 90 degrees and your thigh is parallel to the floor. With your hands at your sides, maintain your gaze and take five full breaths. Lower that leg, turn around (wall on your right now), and repeat with the left leg. Once this becomes easy, try straightening the raised leg and pointing the toe while lifting it as high as possible.

Best **40**+-minute workout:
Strength training

Whenever you have more time to exercise, the best way to spend it is by strength training. Regardless of age, it will tone and build muscle. And since muscle tissue requires more energy to sustain than fat tissue, you'll burn calories even while at rest and lose weight faster. Resistance training also increases bone density, which fights osteoporosis, besides just helping us cope with the physical demands of life. Plus, when done in a circuit with little rest in between exercises, it becomes aerobic.

What follows is a total-body strength workout that uses dumbbells for most exercises and takes 40 minutes or more to complete. Start by doing one set of 8 to 12 repetitions for each exercise at a comfortable pace and with a manageable weight. Once that becomes easy, add more weight, a second or third set of reps, or rest less in between exercises.

Warm up

Do 5 minutes of activity that gets your blood flowing and your muscles moving. Great choices include walking in place, lifting your knees high as you go; walking on a treadmill; peddling on a stationary bike; going up and down stairs; or doing 25 to 50 jumping jacks.

Lunge

- *quadriceps*
- *hamstrings*
- *buttocks*

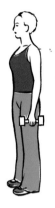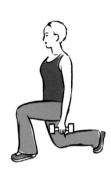

Stand tall with feet hip-width apart and dumbbells at your sides. Take a big step forward with your left foot, keeping your upper body perpendicular to the ground and left knee over the ankle. You'll end up on the ball of your right foot with that knee bent. Hold the lunge for a few seconds, then step back to the start position and repeat with the opposite leg. That's one rep.

Calf raise

- *calves*

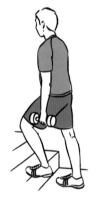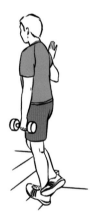

While holding a dumbbell in your left hand at your side, put the toes of your left foot on a bottom stair. Next, while resting your opposite hand on the wall or banister for stability, tuck your right foot behind your left ankle and slowly rise up and down on your toes. Do one set, then switch legs.

Bent-over row

- *low back*
- *shoulders*

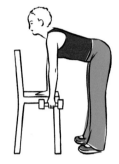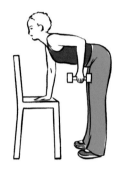

With a dumbbell in your left hand, bend over and rest your right hand on a chair seat. Ground yourself, then pull the weight up toward your underarm while keeping that elbow close to your side. Slowly lower it. That's one rep. After completing your reps on this side, move the weight to the other hand and repeat.

Upright row

- *forearms*
- *shoulders*
- *upper back*

Stand tall with feet hip-width apart and a dumbbell in each hand, palms facing the front of your thighs. Line the weights up along the front of your body until your elbows are parallel to the floor. Pause and return to the start position. That's one rep.

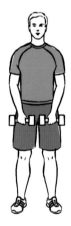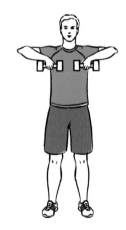

Push-up

- *chest*
- *arms*

Start in a plank position with hands directly beneath shoulders. While keeping your elbows tucked, slowly lower yourself to the floor and then press back up. If this is too difficult, put your knees on the ground.

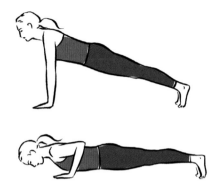

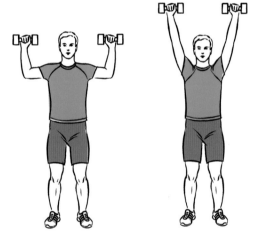

Push press

- *shoulders*
- *arms*

Stand tall with feet hip-width apart while holding a dumbbell in each hand. Raise both arms until the elbows are bent 90 degrees (resembling a goalpost), with palms facing forward and knees bent. Now press both weights overhead as you straighten your legs. Then lower the dumbbells back to the goalpost position as you squat again. That's one rep.

Opposite arm/opposite leg

- *low back*
- *posterior legs*
- *shoulders*

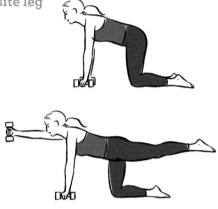

Assume a table position on the floor, with knees directly under hips and each hand grasping a dumbbell (directly under shoulders, palms turned in). Raise and extend your left leg while doing the same with your right arm. Pause for 2 or 3 seconds with that leg and arm parallel to the ground, then lower and repeat on the other side. That's one rep.

Crunch

- *abdominals*

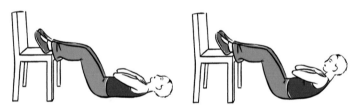

Lie on your back with knees bent and feet on a chair seat. Fold your arms across your chest with fingertips touching opposite shoulders. While keeping your elbows and chin tucked, slowly curl your upper body toward your legs, hold for a few seconds, and then slowly lower down.

Cool down

5 minutes (light stretching)

PERSONAL N●TES

{ How do I waste time, and how can I use that **time better?** }

Cut your
cholesterol, naturally

Cholesterol-lowering drugs are cheap and effective. So why not just pop a daily pill and stop worrying about clogged arteries? If your doctor says you need them, we have no argument. But if it's partly your decision, consider:

▸ *Too many people nowadays address every problem with a pill until their medicine cabinet looks like a CVS shelf. Overmedication is a serious health problem in itself.*

▸ *Not addressing the root causes of high cholesterol, such as a poor diet and/or a sedentary lifestyle puts you at risk of developing other chronic illnesses, like hypertension and diabetes.*

So while swallowing a pill may seem like the simplest solution, you might be making it harder on yourself long-term. Make sense? Good. Now let's begin with the three most effective strategies for managing cholesterol naturally.

Rough up your diet

The number one foodstuff for lowering cholesterol, according to doctors at the Mayo Clinic, is soluble fiber. It reduces the absorption of cholesterol into the blood while targeting its worst component (LDL). There are an overwhelming array of cholesterol-fighting foods and claims, but people with diets highest in fiber reduce their risk of heart disease by nearly a third. The recommended daily allowance for men is 36 grams and for women 28 grams. Doing so will also ensure that you eat more fruits and vegetables, less saturated fat and junk food, and fewer calories overall (because fiber-rich foods fill you up). Oatmeal, kidney beans, apples, pears, barley, and sun-dried plums are all soluble superstars.

Follow this training plan

Although any exercise lends heart and health benefits, there are particular ones that seem to control cholesterol best. The more you work out aerobically, as measured by duration or distance, the better the results. (Intensity doesn't matter as much.) Research also shows that strength training is effective for improving cholesterol profiles (lowers LDL while raising HDL). So combine the two in a weekly program that alternates three days of longer walks, runs, or bike rides at a moderate pace with three days of total-body resistance training. (If you've been sedentary, work up to these levels slowly under the guidance of a doctor and trainer.)

Become less of a man (or woman)

Losing weight—even as little as 5 or 10 pounds—produces beneficial changes in cholesterol. Even better news: If you follow our first two tips, you won't have to do anything extra to achieve this. You'll drop pounds automatically.

POP, POP, POP...

48 ›› Percent of Americans taking at least one prescription drug

20 ›› Americans taking multiple prescription drugs in the last decade

9 out of 10 ›› Number of adults over age 60 taking a prescription drug

1 out of 5 ›› Number of children doing the same

$234 billion ›› Total prescription drug spending in U.S. (2008, latest figure)

3 ›› Rank of cholesterol-lowering meds among all drugs prescribed for adults age 20 to 59. (They're number one for adults 60+)

25 ›› Percent of U.S. adults over age 45 taking a statin

Soothe a
sore muscle

We know, we know. You're constantly being told to exercise more. But when you finally follow through, you feel worse than before. Muscle soreness can leave you hobbling for days. Truth is, if you're that sore, you overdid it. When you exercise again, do a little less and progress gradually from week to week. Meanwhile, you need relief. Here's how to provide it.

Be proud of yourself
If you exercised yesterday and your muscles are mildly sore today, that means you had a productive workout. Muscles require a small degree of damage in order to grow and develop. "If you jog the same two miles at the same pace day after day, you will never become faster or stronger," explains Gabe Mirkin, MD. "All improvement in any muscle function comes from stressing and recovering."

Lactic acid has nothing to do with it
Experts used to think that this caustic substance built up in the muscle during exercise and caused the resulting soreness. But that's not the case, says Dr. Mirkin, who is certified by the American Board of Sports Medicine. It's actually damage to the muscle fibers themselves that's the source of the ache. Biopsies reveal actual bleeding in the muscle tissue.

Pass up the painkillers
Most people reach immediately for ibuprofen and other non-steroidal anti-inflammatories (NSAIDs) when muscle soreness strikes. But there's conflicting evidence as to how helpful these are after exercise. So unless the ache is severe, it might be better to just tough it out.

Ice the inflammation

To help soothe the soreness, cut 1-inch (3-cm) slits in a few old tennis balls, fill them about 75 percent with water, and freeze. They're great for rolling over muscles to reduce inflammation, plus their furry surface prevents skin irritation.

Pop some polyphenols

These antioxidants, which are prevalent in fruits, vegetables, whole wheat, and legumes, have recently been found to reduce muscle inflammation and its resulting tenderness. In fact, they appear to work better than NSAIDs. Studies with concentrated cherry gel and one study with non-alcoholic wheat beer showed significant positive effects.

Take it easy the next few days

Depending on how tender your muscles feel, either rest entirely or exercise lightly. All aches should be gone before working out hard again. Incidentally, Dr. Mirkin says stretching muscles after exercise won't prevent soreness because contracted muscle fibers are not to blame.

GET RID OF A SIDE STITCH These sharp pains are caused by a spasm in the diaphragm muscle or its surrounding tissue. To prevent it, avoid eating a couple hours prior to exercising. If one hits, try one or both of these remedies to get relief quick:

▸▸ **Give yourself the fingers:** Press two fingers up and in toward the hurt just below the ribs and take deep breaths. This should relax the spasm.

▸▸ **Stretch that side:** Stand and raise your right arm overhead (if the stitch is on the right side) and bend to the left. If the stitch is on the opposite side, do the reverse.

Lower your cancer risk

We're not going to dwell on the obvious. Avoiding tobacco, losing weight, exercising regularly, wearing sunscreen, getting recommended tests, and eating lots of whole foods are all proven cancer fighters. This, you should already know. Here are some highly effective strategies based on the latest research that you may underestimate or not be aware of at all.

Update your family history
Your doctor will always ask if there have been any changes in your health since your last visit. Answer this question *broadly,* letting him know if any immediate family members have recently been diagnosed with a disease. Knowing if a first- or second-degree relative has breast or colon cancer, for instance, will help him better gauge your risk and may affect the screenings he recommends.

Follow the rub on sunscreens
After years of lax oversight, the FDA is cracking down. To prevent skin cancer, it recommends using only products labeled "broad spectrum" with an SPF of 15 (or greater) and reapplying as directed. (The terms "waterproof" and "sweatproof" have been banned as misleading.) The feds are also evaluating aerosol sunscreens for effectiveness and nanoparticles of ingredients like zinc and titanium oxide for safety. Stay up to date at cancer.org.

Consider the wonder drug
In a study tracking more than 25,000 patients, those taking a daily low-dose aspirin had a 21 percent lower risk of dying from cancer than those who didn't swallow one. More specifically, rates of lung cancer in the group dropped 30 percent, colorectal cancer 40 percent, and esophageal cancer 60 percent. Consult

with your doctor first, however, since aspirin can cause stomach bleeding and other problems.

Trim your body fat

We know we promised not to belabor the obvious, but half of all Americans aren't aware that obesity is responsible for 100,000 new cases of cancer in the United States each year. Body fat promotes cancer by raising estrogen levels, interfering with insulin production, and causing chronic inflammation. Heavy women are 62 percent more at risk; their male counterparts 52 percent.

Filter your water

One of the top recommendations of the President's Cancer Panel, which recently examined environmental risk factors for cancer, was to filter your home tap or well water. This reduces potential carcinogenic exposure and is better than drinking the bottled stuff, the report concludes. *Consumer Reports* reviews the latest models periodically.

Bookmark this site

If you have a family history of cancer or if avoiding it is a health priority, the website of the American Cancer Society (cancer.org) is an indispensable resource. In researching this book, we visited hundreds of health sites, and it is among the most comprehensive, authoritative, and helpful. The "In the News" section is particularly great for summarizing the latest studies in layman's terms.

Don't get blindsided by
sight problems

We worry that a heart attack or arthritis will compromise our senior years, but one-third of us will have our independence severely curtailed by something we rarely even consider. Vision loss or blindness from cataracts, diabetic retinopathy, glaucoma, and macular degeneration is forecast to rise 50 percent by 2020. This is partially due to Americans living longer, but also to many of us just taking our eyesight for granted. Not anymore.

Follow this checkup schedule
Most vision problems can be managed or corrected if diagnosed early. In your 40s, 50s, and early 60s, you should have a complete eye exam every two to four years. After age 65 it should be annual. Seniors who haven't had an eye exam in more than three years may be eligible for a free one (visit eyecaremerica.org).

Avoid or reverse diabetes
People with diabetes (types 1 and 2) are 25 times more likely to lose their vision than people without the disease. See page 118 for our best tips on preventing diabetes. Or if you've already been diagnosed, consider this additional incentive to manage it more stringently.

Go Hollywood
The sun's UV rays can fry your eyes just as they can your skin. To avoid corneal sunburn, wear wraparound-style sunglasses that block 100 percent of all UV light. You can also get UV coatings on contact lenses.

Eat more kale than carrots

Mom was half right: Carrots do contain lots of eye-nourishing nutrients. But the best food for your vision is dark green leafy vegetables, like spinach, Swiss chard, and especially kale. They contain lutein and zeaxanthin, antioxidants that may even reduce the progression of age-related macular degeneration. If you're not a fan of their taste, toss a cup into stir-fry, soups, and pasta sauces, where you'll barely notice them. Overall, the more fruits, vegetables, and whole foods in your diet, the healthier you're eyes will be.

Wear eye protection

Most eye injuries don't occur on assembly lines or sports fields. They happen doing everyday household chores. Buy a few pairs of ANSI-approved (that's the American National Standards Institute) goggles at the hardware store and put a set in the garage, basement, kitchen, and wherever they'll be handy.

See into the future

To actually experience what it's like to have cataracts, diabetic retinopathy, glaucoma, or macular degeneration, visit eyecareamerica.org and click on "eye disease simulators." If this doesn't prompt you to take better care of your peepers, nothing will.

DO YOU HAVE MACULAR DEGENERATION? Go to macular.org/chart.html for a test. It is called Amsler's Grid. To use it, hold a printout of the page at arm's length and eye level (with reading glasses on, if necessary). Cover one eye and gaze at the center dot, then repeat with the opposite eye. If any lines are distorted or missing, see an eye doctor for further testing.

Let your pet
be your doctor

One day in the not-too distant future, you may encounter sniffer dogs in your doctor's office just like you do at the airport. Researchers are finding that certain breeds of dogs can detect cancers (prostate, colon, skin, lung, bowel, breast), sense impending hypoglycemic episodes, and may even be able to warn of seizures (see "Good Boy," on page 125). Although exactly how they do this is unclear, it's believed they can pick out a disease's odor, as well as subtle behavioral changes in people. But you don't have to wait until pooch prevention is perfected. There are other ways you can use a pet to make yourself and your family healthier.

Fitness partner
One of the best ways to get fit and stay fit is to recruit an exercise buddy—someone who'll goad you into working out when you don't feel like it. Well, that buddy doesn't have to be human. An active dog that shows up each morning with leash in mouth is just as difficult to flout.

Stress reducer
Simply petting an animal lowers blood pressure and decreases heart rate. In a classic study of stockbrokers with hypertension, those who took in a dog or cat were better able to handle job pressure.

Heart builder
Dog owners generally have lower levels of triglercerides and male pet owners have lower LDL (bad) cholesterol levels, meaning they have less risk of heart disease. But on a broader level, caring for a pet and seeing an appreciative tail wag encourages feelings of well-being that make people feel happier, better

connected, and perhaps most important, unconditionally loved. In many hospitals and eldercare facilities, service dogs make rounds just like doctors, comforting patients and residents.

Habit breaker

Let's say you want your dog's help to quit smoking. First, use a treat to teach your pet to bark on command when ordering, "Speak!" Once he's mastered this, hold up a pack of cigarettes, give the same command, and then reward him when he cooperates. In no time he'll be barking whenever you reach for your Marlboros, which will hopefully serve as a reminder not to light up. The same strategy can be creatively applied to any bad habit you're trying to kick, such as biting nails or wolfing down snacks.

Allergy fighter

Contrary to popular belief, having a furry pet in the house appears to help immunize some kids to allergens and boost their immune systems. However, if your youngster is seriously allergic, buy the cutest, most cuddly stuffed animal you can find. A couple of studies have found that puppy dolls help children better cope with stress. While you're at it, buy one for yourself. No one has to know.

BUT DON'T LET HIM DO THIS Mattress-manufacturer Sealy found that 67 percent of pet owners regularly sleep with their dogs and cats. Thirty-eight percent, however, confessed that their animals were far from perfect sleepers and disturbed their night's rest. Researchers at the Mayo Clinic Sleep Disorders Center found that snoring, especially among dogs, was a common culprit.

Boost your fertility

You might have worried about it happening all through your wanton youth. But now that you're actually trying to have a baby and it's not happening, you're even more anxious. You're not alone. Just over 6 million Americans struggle with infertility each year, and it can be emotionally as well as financially draining. But there are some simple lifestyle changes that can make a big difference. Try these before seeing a specialist.

Calculate your baby-making index

You've probably heard of BMI (body mass index) as a gauge for whether you're under- or overweight. But it can also be viewed as the baby-making index because body fat plays a critical role in reproduction. Go to nhlbisupport.com/bmi and calculate BMI for you and your partner. If one or both of you are below or above the norm, your fertility is being compromised. If you're having problems conceiving, address any weight issues first.

Clear the air

Women who smoke have a 60 percent greater risk of infertility than those who don't. And although smoking's effect on the male reproductive system doesn't appear to be as dramatic, if a spouse puffs, secondhand smoke is nearly as destructive. Fortunately, quitting has immediate benefits, with fertility usually returning to normal within a year.

Don't go to extremes

Whether it's alcohol, caffeine, or even exercise, your new mantra should be moderation. Consuming more than two alcoholic drinks or more than five cups of coffee (totaling 500 mg of caffeine) daily has been shown to decrease fertility in women. Likewise, exercising for more than an hour per day can interfere with ovulation.

Give lubes the slip

For those times when you need a vaginal lubricant, the American Society for Reproductive Medicine recommends mineral or canola oil. Commercially available lubes such as KY Jelly, Astroglide, and Touch inhibit sperm motility.

Scrutinize that scrotum

A common cause of male infertility is varicoceles—dilated or varicose veins in the scrotum. Forty percent of men experiencing infertility have them. After a warm shower, when things are most relaxed, check for what will feel like a small ball of worms or even spaghetti in either sack. A doctor should check anything suspicious.

Make love more often

Many couple believe that frequent ejaculation decreases sperm count. Not so. Reproductive efficiency, as those romantic researchers like to call it, is highest when intercourse occurs every one to two days. Incidentally, no one sexual position is better (or worse) for conception than another, but of course, you're free to continue the research.

Relax

That's right. Resign yourself to a kidless life if that's what it takes to notch down the pressure. Stress plays havoc with fertility, too.

A TRUE ROMANTIC MEAL Although research is continuing, there appears to be certain foods that boost fertility. So we've combined them into one meal. Don't forget the candles.

Appetizer

▸▸ **Oysters:** Zinc promotes semen production and ovulation.

Entrée

▸▸ **Salmon:** Omega-3 fatty acids increase blood flow to the uterus.

▸▸ **Steamed broccoli:** foods high in vitamin C increase fertility.

▸▸ **Lentils:** beans have folate, which increases sperm count and density.

▸▸ **Wine:** Time to conceive for women who have an occasional glass is shorter than for teetotalers, according to a Danish study.

Dessert

▸▸ **Ice cream:** A twice-weekly half-cup serving of full-fat dairy increased the odds of pregnancy in a study of 19,000 nurses.

PERSONAL NOTES

What can I do to make my **relationship** healthier for me?

Soothe a sore throat

Sore throats are worrisome because their cause is often unclear. Is it a sign of impeding cold or flu, or is it the result of yet another night of karaoke you hope didn't make it onto YouTube? Or maybe it's something worse—like strep, mono, or even the throat cancer that actor Michael Douglas had. Before you stress out, here's some diagnostic advice that's easy to swallow.

Open wide and take a photo
To get a rough idea of what's going on in there, snap a shot of the back of your throat. At the very least, it'll make an interesting addition to your Facebook page. And if things look angry and inflamed, you'll have confirmed an infection.

Wait out a virus
The same viruses that trigger colds and flu cause most sore throats. So if you also have the sniffles and your throat is just mildly sore, the best treatment is to gargle, sip liquids, suck lozenges, and let the bug run its course (usually five to seven days). *Don't* take antibiotics; they do nothing for viral infections. (Note: If these symptoms persist and are accompanied by swollen lymph nodes in the neck and armpits, plus general fatigue and low-grade fever, see a doctor, because it could be mono.)

Test for bacteria
If your sore throat is severe with a high fever and swollen glands or lasts beyond a week, the infection could be bacterial. This is more serious and needs a doctor's attention. The good news is that bacterial infections do respond to antibiotics.

Don't mess around with recurrent ones
If you're regularly plagued by a sore throat, it could be tonsillitis or, if the symptoms are seasonal, allergy related. Even worse,

if a sore throat keeps returning, get checked for throat cancer. There's one type—oropharyngeal cancer—that affects both smokers and nonsmokers and is linked to the same virus (HPV) that's linked to cervical cancer. It's on the rise.

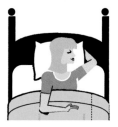

Revamp your bedroom

When there are no visible signs of inflammation or other symptoms but your throat is scratchy in the morning, it could be a simple case of sleeping with your mouth open or inhaling dry air. Try raising your head above your stomach with a more supportive pillow or by putting bricks under the two top bedposts. If that doesn't work, put a humidifier in the room.

A GAGGLE OF GARGLES Gargling is one of the oldest and most effective home remedies for soothing a sore throat. Everyone from Mom to the Mayo Clinic endorses various concoctions. Experiment with these to find the one that works best for you:

▸▸ **The Classic:** 1 cup warm water with 1/4 teaspoon salt.

▸▸ **The Classic Plus:** Same as above but with an additional tablespoon of Listerine (for germ killing).

▸▸ **The New Favorite:** 1 cup warm water with 1 teaspoon lemon juice. (The astringent juice shrinks swollen tissue, while the acid fights viruses and bacteria.)

▸▸ **The No Hassle:** "Simply Gargle" single-dose packets for sale at drugstores. (Each one contains 0.4 ounces of premixed water, salt, vitamin C, and other sore-throat soothers.)

▸▸ **The Nightcap:** 1/2 cup warm water, juice from 1/2 lemon, 1 teaspoon powdered ginger, 1 teaspoon honey. (Coats the throat and has mild antibacterial properties.)

Make these health moves in
your
60s (and beyond)

What	When
Routine checks/exams	
Complete physical	Every 1—3 years
Blood pressure	Every 6 months
Cholesterol	Every 2 years
Blood glucose	Every 3 years
Eyesight	Biannually < 65; Annually > 65
Teeth	Twice yearly
Hearing	Every 3 years
Body mass index (BMI)	Every 6 months
Skin cancer	Annually
Prostate specific antigen (PSA)	Periodically; ask your doctor
Digital rectal	Annually
Fecal occult blood	Annually
Sigmoidoscopy	Every 5 years
Colonoscopy	Once per decade
Bone density	Periodically *(if at risk; ask your doctor)*
Mammogram	Annually
Pelvic exam/Pap test	Every 2 to 3 years < 65, *then ask doctor*
Thyroid	Every 5 years

Health... The Reader's Digest VERSION

Some very smart people spend their entire lives saving for their senior years, only to find that when the time arrives, health is the new wealth. Hopefully, your personal portfolio is robust with this investment and your interest is compounding. But even if it isn't, there's still plenty of time to catch up. Remember: Age alone doesn't cause you to become sick or feeble, Decline is a function of how you choose to live.

Inoculations

Influenza	Annually
Pneumonia	Once per lifetime > 65
Shingles	Once per lifetime
Tetanus-diphtheria	Once per decade
Others	If missed in prior decades (see page 42)

General

Volunteer.	Giving back lowers risk of death.
Make more friends.	Social support boosts immunity.
Lift weights/eat protein.	Fights muscle/strength loss.
Go back to school.	Learning promotes brain growth.

Find allergy relief

First, look on the bright side. Your allergies to pollen, dust, mold, pet dander, or whatever else is making you miserable could mean you have a lower risk of brain tumors and cancer. Scientists theorize that since allergies are caused by an overactive immune system, such a SWAT-like response could ward off other cellular invaders as well. So when the sniffles strike, keep that in mind. In the meantime...

Hit the bedroom hard

Since you spend about a third of your life sleeping, direct most of your home allergy-proofing efforts here. Besides regular cleaning, get rid of carpeting and heavy drapery that can harbor allergens, keep windows and doors closed (especially to a damp bathroom), and move Fluffy out. (We're talking about your pet, not your spouse.) Also, zip pillows, mattress, and box spring inside allergen-impermeable covers. And if you can't launder all the bedding weekly (in 130°F/54°C water as recommended), at least wash the pillowcases, since your face presses against them all night.

Take better care of your hair

Your do is out in the world all day collecting Lord knows what, so don't go to bed without washing it. (Or bring back the nightcap—nonalcoholic.) Similarly, one study found that men who scrubbed their mustache twice daily with liquid soap needed fewer antihistamines and decongestants.

Check the probability of nose precipitation

You plan your activities around the weather, so why not pay similar attention to the allergy forecast? You'll find pollen and mold counts on most weather websites and at the National Allergy Bureau (aaaai.org). On days when things look threatening, limit outdoor activities and keep all windows closed.

Try one of these

Claritin was the most recommended over-the-counter antihistamine by pharmacists in a recent survey, and its generic form (loratadine) was named a "best buy" by *Consumer Reports Health.* It causes less drowsiness than traditional antihistamines, and only one dose is needed every 12 or 24 hours. (Its cousin, Claritin-D, contains an additional decongestant.) Antihistamines work best, though, when taken *before* allergy symptoms hit.

Pinpoint the problem

Most people have only a vague sense of what's causing their allergies. To find out for sure so you can fight back properly, make an appointment with a board-certified allergist (look for the "find the allergist" link at acaai.org). She'll conduct skin and/or blood tests to pinpoint the source, then recommend treatments, one of which may be immunotherapy. This involves giving extracts of the allergen by injection or via drops under the tongue (sublingual) to provoke the body's immune system. It can take months or even years to work, but if it allows you to garden, bicycle, or snuggle with Fluffy, then isn't it worth it?

IT COULD BE WORSE: 5 REALLY WEIRD ALLERGIES

▸▸ **Kissing:** Some people with food allergies can have a reaction after smooching someone who ate what they're sensitive to.

▸▸ **Sex:** It's possible to be allergic to spermicides, lubricants, latex, and even semen.

▸▸ **Talking on the phone:** This allergy stems from prolonged exposure to the nickel inside most mobile phones. It causes itching in the cheeks and jaw.

▸▸ **Tattoos:** The color pigments can trigger a reaction.

▸▸ **Wine:** Newly discovered "glycoproteins" appear to be the culprit.

End back pain forever

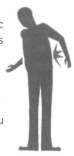

Low back pain is the most common type of chronic pain, plaguing almost twice as many people as the next biggest hurt (headaches). Eighty percent of adults will suffer a sore back at some point in life. Fortunately, most cases won't require hospitalization or surgery and can be managed and even cured with lifestyle changes. Here are some little things you can do to make your spine smile.

Clean out your purse

One sneaky cause of chronic back pain is overloaded handbags, backpacks, and briefcases. Hanging a heavy weight off one side of your body (when you're in heels, no less) stresses your entire skeleton as it tries to compensate. Weigh your bag on the bathroom scale. If it's more than 10 percent of your body weight, pare it down (or buy a lighter one at Coach).

Carry less cash

Hey, big spender, sitting on a fat wallet all day twists the spine and compresses nerves in the buttocks and leg. Sciatica is the inflammation of those nerves. This problem is so common among men that it has a clinical name: wallet neuropathy.

Reach for heat before pills

When low back pain strikes, try treating it with ThermaCare HeatWraps rather than ibuprofen or acetaminophen. These wearable pads provide 104°F (40°C) heat for up to eight hours. A study published in *Spine* (what, you don't subscribe?) found they supply more relief than the maximum dose of nonprescription pain relievers and have longer-lasting effects. By increasing blood flow to the sore spot, they promote healing and mobility. Staying active is important because bed rest appears to make back pain worse.

Get some pants tailored

This is a quick and inexpensive way to determine if one of your legs is shorter than the other. Nobody's perfect, and any discrepancy greater than three-fifths of an inch could affect your back. If the tailor detects a difference, put a Dr. Scholl's–type lift in your shoe or consult a podiatrist about custom inserts.

Tune up your body mechanics

When standing for any length of time, get in the habit of keeping one foot in front of the other. When sitting at your desk or on a long flight, put something under your feet so your knees are slightly higher than your hips. Both ease pressure on the lower back.

Assume the position

The best sleeping position if you have a bad back is on your side with a pillow tucked between bent knees. Sleeping faceup or down arches the spine and prevents it from fully relaxing. To keep from rolling onto your back or belly while you're unconscious, duct-tape a golf ball to the front and rear of your nightshirt. Chances are, you'll wake up feeling above par.

LET'S ROLL A recent study found the benefits of regular Swedish massage to be "about as strong as medications, acupuncture, exercise, and yoga" for treating back pain. But unless you're married to someone named Rolf or Inga, it may be an indulgence that's too expensive to afford. Enter the high-density foam roller, a self-massage tool that's especially effective at working out kinks and promoting blood flow to the lower back. Simply roll around on top of it using your body weight for pressure. You can find foam rollers at any sporting goods store or visit tptherapy.com/shop/smrt-core-products.html to check out a ridged model called The Grid.

Heal yourself
with mind power

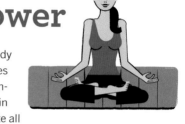

Although we tend to view body and mind as separate entities (thank you, all you Playboy bunnies), the two are intertwined in ways that medical science, despite all its progress, is just fathoming. But that needn't stop you from experimenting. Whether you're out to muster your defenses for flu season or manage a chronic disease in yourself or a loved one, here's how to potentially recruit your greatest ally.

Learn the relaxation response
Harvard Medical School professor Herbert Benson, MD, estimates that 60 to 90 percent of doctor visits are linked in some way to stress. So it follows that if you can learn to manage stress better, your health will automatically improve. The key, he says, is eliciting the "relaxation response." This is a deep but conscious state of rest that lowers metabolism, heart rate, respiration, blood pressure, and muscle tension—all of which promotes healing and well-being. To learn it, sit quietly in a comfortable position, close your eyes, and breathe slowly and naturally. Once you're relaxed, start repeating a personally meaningful word or phrase (such as love, peace, Hail Mary full of grace, John Lennon ...). Continue for 10 to 20 minutes, practicing twice daily. You should eventually feel more balanced.

Pop a placebo
You've no doubt heard about participants in clinical trials who unknowingly got sugar pills yet experienced measurable positive effects. This is the power of belief at work. In fact, the American Cancer Society states that while placebos do not act on disease, "they seem to have an effect in 1 out of 3 patients."

Although you can't evoke a placebo effect in yourself (because you know what's being done), if you're looking to ease the suffering of a chronically ill relative or friend, consider asking their doctor to "prescribe" a placebo. About half of American doctors surveyed admitted to doing this in some situations.

Say your prayers

There is some research supporting the long-held belief that praying, whether for yourself or others, can positively influence health. On one level, petitioning a Higher Power to intercede on your behalf counters feelings of stress and powerlessness. On another, being prayed for by others reinforces your connection with family and community, which can be empowering and actually speed healing. It doesn't even matter if the praying is done in church. A study of breast cancer patients who prayed in online support groups found evidence of lower negativity and higher well-being.

Be a little more optimistic

Having a positive outlook on life has been shown to lower the risk of heart disease and stroke, protect against breast cancer, and reduce the odds of dying from any cause compared to people who are more pessimistic. There now, isn't that terrific news?

MEDITATE WHILE YOU MOVE If sitting quietly trying to evoke the relaxation response drives you nuts, take a different approach: Do it while exercising. Instead of focusing on a word or phrase, let the movement be your mantra. For example, when walking outside or on a treadmill, bring your attention to each footfall—left/right/left/right. In other words, let its sound and feel be your metronome. This is what's known as "mindful exercise." After a while it can put you in a zone that is just as rejuvenating and nourishing as conventional meditation.

PROJECT STAFF
Writer Joe Kita
Project Editors Neil Wertheimer, Dolores York
Fact Checking Evelyn Bollert
Copy Editor Barbara Booth
Consulting Art Director Elizabeth Tunnicliffe
Interior Design Vertigo Design LLC
Cover Design Jennifer Tokarski
Illustrations Scotty Reifsnyder
Fitness Illustrations Nicole Kaufman

Reader's Digest **Magazine**
   Global Editor in Chief Peggy Northrop
   Creative Director Robert Newman
   Vice President, General Manager, Reader's Digest Media Marilynn Jacobs
   Executive Editor Tom Prince
   Managing Editor Ann Powell
   Senior Editor Beth Dreher
   General Manager, rd.com Matt Goldenberg
   Assistant Managing Editor Paul Silverman
   Copy Editor Janice K. Bryant
   Editorial Assistant Elizabeth Kelly

READER'S DIGEST BOOKS AND HOME ENTERTAINMENT
President and Publisher Harold Clarke
Associate Publisher Rosanne McManus
Senior Art Director George McKeon
Director, Sales and Marketing Stacey Ashton

THE READER'S DIGEST ASSOCIATION, INC.
President and Chief Executive Officer Robert E. Guth
President, Reader's Digest North America Dan Lagani
President, Reader's Digest International Dawn Zier

The Reader's Digest VERSION

For more information, visit Reader's Digest online at rd.com

Also available from Reader's Digest

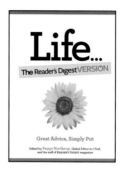

Life...The Reader's Digest VERSION

Great Advice, Simply Put

Edited by Peggy Northrop, Global Editor-in-Chief, and the staff of READER'S DIGEST magazine

With more to do and less time to do it in than ever before, **LIFE...The Reader's Digest Version** gets straight to the answers, presenting essential advice to help you be better and do better. From the big stuff, such as how to console someone, to the small stuff, such as how to give a toast, here are the most practical ways to succeed at more than 70 of life's most common yet confounding tasks.

Reader's Digest books can be purchased through retail and online stores. For more information or to order books, call 1-800-788-6262.

eep great tonight (and every nigh
me health traps • Brave a craving
permarket shopper • Best 10-m
nd your ideal exercise • Beat fatigu
erapist • Decide if organic is wort
ake these health moves in your 2
od-borne illness • Boost your i
Run/walks • Find the right diet
overseas • health emergency • Ma
sess the health of your workplace
ting for you? • Finding solutic
oring • Tell if it's impotency or b
ur 50s • Prevent diabetes • Beat d
r skin cancer • Get rid of a cold
75 percent • Flatten your stor
alth • Managing the system • Fin
sts • Best 20-minute workout